A Case-Based Approach to Neck Pain

Michael Harbus • Grant Cooper
Joseph E. Herrera • Zinovy Meyler
Marco Funiciello
Editors

A Case-Based Approach to Neck Pain

A Pocket Guide to Pathology, Diagnosis and Management

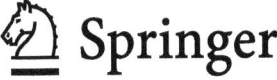 Springer

Editors
Michael Harbus
Physical Medicine
and Rehabilitation
Mount Sinai Hospital
New York, NY, USA

Joseph E. Herrera
Department of Rehabilitation Medicine
Mount Sinai Hospital
New York, NY, USA

Marco Funiciello
Princeton Spine and Joint Center
Princeton, NJ, USA

Grant Cooper
Princeton Spine and Joint Center
Princeton, NJ, USA

Zinovy Meyler
Princeton Spine and Joint Center
Princeton, NJ, USA

ISBN 978-3-031-17307-3   ISBN 978-3-031-17308-0 (eBook)
https://doi.org/10.1007/978-3-031-17308-0

© The Editor(s) (if applicable) and The Author(s), under exclusive license to Springer Nature Switzerland AG 2022
This work is subject to copyright. All rights are solely and exclusively licensed by the Publisher, whether the whole or part of the material is concerned, specifically the rights of translation, reprinting, reuse of illustrations, recitation, broadcasting, reproduction on microfilms or in any other physical way, and transmission or information storage and retrieval, electronic adaptation, computer software, or by similar or dissimilar methodology now known or hereafter developed.
The use of general descriptive names, registered names, trademarks, service marks, etc. in this publication does not imply, even in the absence of a specific statement, that such names are exempt from the relevant protective laws and regulations and therefore free for general use.
The publisher, the authors, and the editors are safe to assume that the advice and information in this book are believed to be true and accurate at the date of publication. Neither the publisher nor the authors or the editors give a warranty, expressed or implied, with respect to the material contained herein or for any errors or omissions that may have been made. The publisher remains neutral with regard to jurisdictional claims in published maps and institutional affiliations.

This Springer imprint is published by the registered company Springer Nature Switzerland AG
The registered company address is: Gewerbestrasse 11, 6330 Cham, Switzerland

For Stephanie, Ellen, Fred, Carolyn and Milton

Michael Harbus

For Ana, Mila, Lara, Luka, Twinkle and Lili

Grant Cooper

For my parents Anna and Mark, they serve as role models and shaped my character; their many sacrifices were aimed to provide me with opportunities in life.

Zinovy Meyler

To my loving wife Bonnie and our beautiful children Antonella, Juliana, Mia and Gianluca, thank you for your love, patience and never-ending dedication to reading and a heartfelt thank you to my parents who made a lot of pizza to help me with medical school bills.

Marco Funiciello

Preface

This book is designed to serve as a reference for students and healthcare providers who treat neck pain. Neck pain is a common presenting complaint of patients who visit providers who treat musculoskeletal conditions. As with many musculoskeletal complaints, there is significant overlap in the presentation of many of the pathologies that cause neck pain, which can create challenges in arriving at an accurate diagnosis based on a patient's history and physical exam.

The book provides an overview of the most common causes of neck pain including strains, sprains, facet-mediated pain, radiculopathies and discogenic pain, and it delves into the diagnosis and treatment for these commonly seen conditions. The book presents the anatomy, pathophysiology, presentation, diagnostic work-up and evidence-based treatment plans for common causes of neck pain in an easily accessible manner. By doing so, we hope that it will enable its readers to provide more accurate diagnosis and effective treatments for their patients.

Ultimately, this book aims to guide providers from multiple specialties and disciplines—including physical therapists, primary care physicians, physiatrists and spine surgeons—in their approach when treating patients who present with neck pain.

New York, NY, USA	Michael Harbus
Princeton, NJ, USA	Grant Cooper
New York, NY, USA	Joseph E. Herrera
Princeton, NJ, USA	Zinovy Meyler
Princeton, NJ, USA	Marco Funiciello

Acknowledgements

I want to thank my wife, Stephanie, for her endless generosity and understanding; my parents, Ellen and Fred, for their selflessness, and for being the best role models I could ask for; my sister, Carolyn, for always being a source of advice and support; and my grandparents, who taught me immeasurable amounts about hard work, family and balance. I would also like to thank my co-editors whose guidance made this book possible.
Michael Harbus

It has been a pleasure to collaborate on this book. I want to first thank my co-editors and all of the amazing authors who worked so hard to make this book a reality. Thank you to my colleagues at Princeton Spine and Joint Center for continuing to push, nurture and challenge me. And thank you to my family, Ana, Mila, Lara, Luka, Twinkle and Lili for putting up with me when I disappear into the study to write.
Grant Cooper

I would like to thank my amazing family, Sandra, Alex, Mikhayla and Andrew for all of their continued love and support through this journey. Thank you of course to my long-time friend, colleague and co-editor on this and so many other projects, Dr. Grant Cooper. Thank you to all of our fantastic authors and other editors who came together to make this book a success.
Joseph E. Herrera, DO, FAAPMR

I would like to thank all of the great authors contributing to this book, as well as my co-editors. I would also like to thank all friends and colleagues for their support and camaraderie. I would like to extend special gratitude to Ana and Grant for wearing so many hats in my life including those of colleagues, pillars of support, advisors and advocates and for transcending friendship into what feels like family.

Zinovy Meyler

A special thank you to my patients, my greatest teachers. Thank you to our book's co-contributors, without your help this work would not have been possible and to my colleagues at Princeton Spine and Joint Center who continue to help inspire my passion for medicine.

Thank you,

Marco Funiciello

Contents

1. **Cervical Anatomy** 1
   Craig Silverberg, Marya Ghazzi, and Michael Harbus

2. **Cervical Strains and Sprains** 17
   Michael Harbus and Leili Shahgholi

3. **Facet Joint Pain** 25
   Chandni Patel

4. **Discogenic Pain** 37
   Caroline Varlotta

5. **Cervical Radiculopathy** 55
   Jonathan Lee, Michael Harbus, and Carley Trentman

6. **Cervical Myelopathy** 65
   Toqa Afifi, Karolina Zektser, and Aditya Raghunandan

7. **Sports Trauma and Fractures** 95
   Rebecca Freedman and Irene Kalbian

8. **Rheumatologic Causes of Neck Pain** 119
   German Valdez

9. **Case Studies** 127
   Caroline Varlotta

Index 139

Cervical Anatomy

Craig Silverberg, Marya Ghazzi, and Michael Harbus

Introduction

This chapter provides an overview of the structures that make up the neck. Included among these structures are the cervical vertebrae, soft tissue structures, muscles, and vascular and lymphatic structures. Additionally, a detailed review of the neurological structures of the central nervous system, the peripheral nervous system, and the autonomic nervous system that reside in the neck is provided. The anatomical groundwork that is established in this chapter will allow for an enhanced understanding of the pathological conditions discussed throughout the book.

C. Silverberg · M. Harbus (✉)
Department of Rehabilitation and Human Performance, Icahn School of Medicine at Mount Sinai, New York, NY, USA
e-mail: Craig.Silverberg@mountsinai.org

M. Ghazzi
Philadelphia College of Osteopathic Medicine, Philadelphia, PA, USA
e-mail: mg270648@pcom.edu

© The Author(s), under exclusive license to Springer Nature Switzerland AG 2022
M. Harbus et al. (eds.), *A Case-Based Approach to Neck Pain*, https://doi.org/10.1007/978-3-031-17308-0_1

Vertebrae

The cervical spine is the most superior portion of the vertebral column, located between the cranium and thoracic spine. There are seven cervical vertebrae referred to as C1–C7. The cervical spine is divided into two major segments: the craniocervical junction (CCJ) and the subaxial spine. The CCJ includes the occiput and the two most cranial cervical vertebrae known as the atlas (C1) and the axis (C2). The subaxial spine contains the remaining cervical vertebrae (C3–C7) [1].

The atlas (C1) is a ring-like, kidney-shaped bone that lacks a spinous process and consists of two lateral masses connected by anterior and posterior arches. Its concave superior articular facets receive the occipital condyles. The axis (C2) contains the dens, also known as the odontoid process, which extends superiorly from the anterior portion of the vertebra. The dens articulates with the anterior arch of C1, forming the atlanto-axial joint. This joint allows for rotation of the head independently of the torso [1].

The average range of motion of the cervical spine consists of: 65 degrees of flexion, 40 degrees of extension, 35 degrees of lateral flexion, and 35 degrees of rotation. Among these numbers, the atlanto-occipital joint is responsible for 20 degrees of flexion, 10 degrees of extension, and 5 degrees of lateral flexion. The atlanto-axial joint is responsible for 35 degrees of rotation [1].

The subaxial spine contains the five most caudal cervical vertebrae (C3–C7). The four typical cervical vertebrae (C3–C6) have the following characteristics [1]:

- The vertebral body is small and longer from side to side than anteroposteriorly; the superior surface is concave, and the inferior surface is convex.
- The vertebral foramen is large and triangular.
- The superior facets of the articular processes are directed superoposteriorly, and the inferior facets are directed inferoposteriorly.

1 Cervical Anatomy

The atypical cervical vertebrae of the subaxial spine, C7, have a singular and very long spinous process. This is the first spinous process that is distinctly palpable through the skin, known as the prominens, which closely resembles the thoracic vertebrae.

The cervical transverse processes consist of an anterior and a posterior bar, which terminate laterally in two small tubercles (anterior and posterior tubercles). These bars encompass the transverse foramen. Injury to this part of the cervical spine can be very severe, as the transverse foramen gives passage to the vertebral artery, vein, and sympathetic plexus to ascend from the C6 to the C1 level (Fig. 1.1).

The cervical spine is responsible for supporting the weight of the cranium, protecting the spinal cord extending from the brain, and cushioning loads while allowing for various movements of

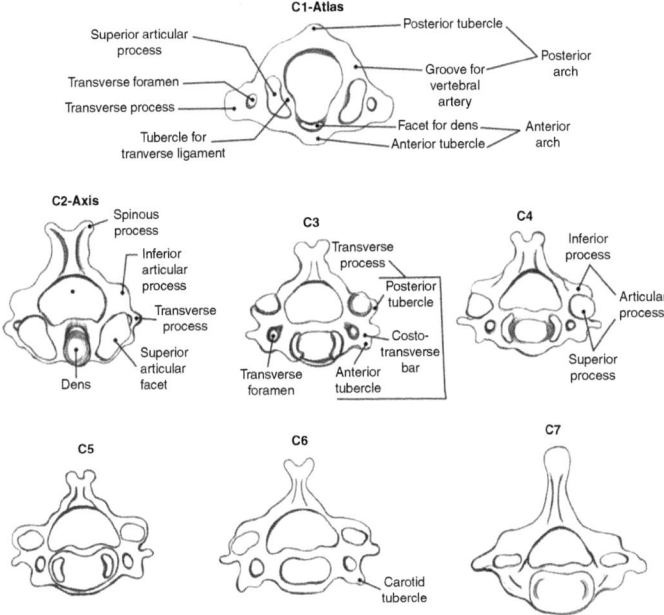

Fig. 1.1 Axial views of cervical vertebrae C1–C7 (From [8])

the head and neck. There are eight pairs of cervical nerves that emerge from the spinal cord superior to their corresponding vertebrae, except for C8 that exits inferiorly to the C7 vertebra. This is unique compared to the thoracic and lumbar nerves which exit below their corresponding vertebrae [1, 2].

The hyoid bone lies in the anterior part of the neck at the level of the C3 vertebra in the angle between the mandible and the thyroid cartilage. The hyoid is suspended by muscles that connect it to the mandible, styloid processes, thyroid cartilage, manubrium of the sternum, and scapulae. The hyoid is unique among bones for its isolation from the remainder of the skeleton. Functionally, the hyoid provides a movable base for the tongue and attachment for the middle part of the pharynx. The hyoid also maintains the patency of the pharynx, required for swallowing and respiration [1].

Soft Tissue

Structures in the neck are surrounded by a layer of subcutaneous tissue (superficial fascia) and are compartmentalized by layers of deep cervical fascia. The cervical subcutaneous tissue contains cutaneous nerves, blood and lymphatic vessels, superficial lymph nodes, and variable amounts of fat. Anterolaterally, it contains the platysma. The platysma is a broad, thin sheet of muscle in the subcutaneous tissue of the neck that tenses the skin, producing vertical skin ridges and releasing pressure on the superficial veins. It is innervated by the cervical branch of the facial nerve, CN VII. Damage to this branch can cause paralysis of the platysma causing skin to fall away from the neck in slack folds.

The deep cervical fascia supports the cervical viscera (e.g., thyroid gland), muscles, vessels, and deep lymph nodes. The deep cervical fascia surrounds the common carotid arteries, internal jugular veins (IJVs), and vagus nerves to form the carotid sheath. The deep cervical fascia also aligns into natural planes through which tissues may be separated during surgery. In addition, this layer plays a role in limiting the spread of abscesses (collections of pus) resulting from infections to this area [1, 2].

Cervical Anatomy

Muscles

The cervical muscles work together with tendons and ligaments to support and move the neck and head. Common muscles involved with neck pain include the sternocleidomastoid, trapezius, levator scapulae, scalenes, deep cervical flexors, erector spinae, and suboccipital muscles.

The sternocleidomastoid muscle (SCM) attaches to the bony mastoid process on the skull and attaches anteriorly to the sternum and collarbone. The SCM helps in head rotation and tilting the chin and protects the inner structures of the neck. The head rotates away from the side of the contracting SCM. It is innervated by cranial nerve XI, known as the spinal accessory nerve, which is the only cranial nerve to both enter and exit the skull. This nerve also innervates the trapezius muscle.

The trapezius is a large surface muscle that attaches to the medial third of superior nuchal line; external occipital protuberance, *nuchal ligament*, and spinous processes of C7–T12 vertebrae. The trapezius is composed of three parts: descending, ascending, and transverse. The descending part of the trapezius muscle supports the arms. The transverse part retracts the scapula, and the ascending part medially rotates or depresses the scapula. Due to its upper attachment to the occiput and lower cervical *vertebra*, it can easily be injured in patients suffering from *whiplash injury* [1, 2].

The levator scapulae muscle attaches to the transverse processes of the first four cervical vertebrae and descends laterally to insert at the superior angle and medial border of the scapula, between the superior angle and base of the spine of the scapula. It is innervated by the anterior rami of spinal nerves C3 and C4. This muscle helps with lifting the shoulder blade, lateral bending of the neck, and rotation of the head [5, 6].

The scalene muscles are three pairs of lateral neck muscles that connect the mid and lower cervical spine with the top of the rib cage. The anterior and middle scalene muscles attach to the first rib, while the posterior scalene attaches to the second rib. The scalene muscles help with neck flexion and side bending. These muscles are innervated by the anterior branches of the cervical spinal nerves from C3 to C8 (Fig. 1.2).

The deep cervical flexor muscles of the anterior neck consist of the longus colli and longus capitis. These muscles help flex the neck forward as well as stabilize the cervical spine. The longus colli muscle is innervated by the anterior rami of the C2–C6 spinal nerves. The longus capitis muscle is innervated by the anterior rami of the C1–C3 spinal nerves.

The erector spinae are a group of many muscles that attach along the back of the spine. The three main muscles of this group include: spinalis, longissimus, and iliocostalis. In the cervical spine, the erector spinae muscles play key roles in posture, rotation of the neck, and neck extension. These muscles are innervated by the dorsal rami of the first cervical nerve (C1) through the fifth lumbar nerve (L5) [1, 2].

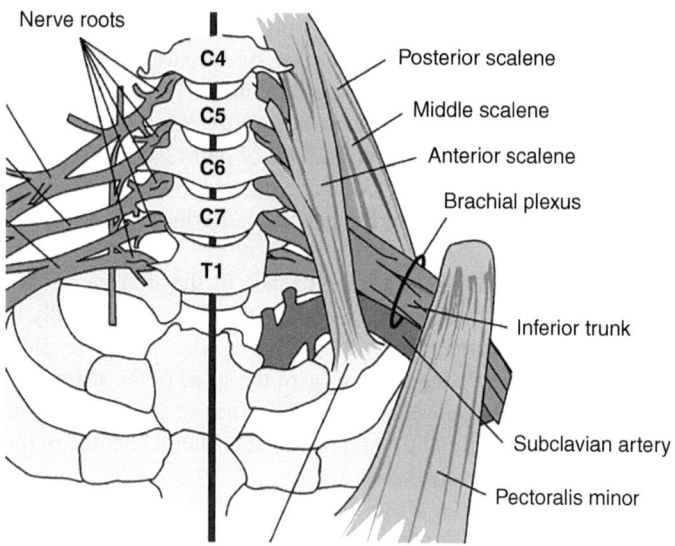

Fig. 1.2 Cervical nerve roots and scalene muscles. (From [8])

1 Cervical Anatomy

The suboccipital muscles are four pairs of small muscles that connect the top of the cervical spine with the base of the skull. These four muscles include the rectus capitis posterior major, rectus capitis posterior minor, obliquus capitis superior, and obliquus capitis inferior. The suboccipitals are needed for head extension and rotation. These muscles are innervated by the suboccipital nerve, also known as the dorsal ramus of the first cervical nerve, which arises from the posterior ramus of the C1 nerve [1, 2].

Spinal Cord

The spinal cord is one of the major neurologic structures of the cervical spine. It emerges from the foramen magnum at the base of the skull and travels to approximately L2. In the cervical spinal cord, the maximum cord circumference is located at C6 and is about 38 mm; this is to accommodate the increased neurologic structures to the upper extremity from the brachial plexus [2]. The spinal cord is made up of an inner gray matter and a surrounding layer of white matter (Fig. 1.3).

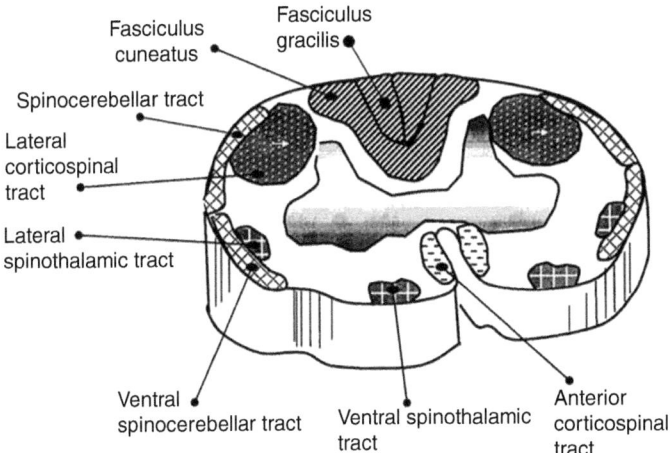

Fig. 1.3 Axial view of the spinal cord. (From [8])

The inner, butterfly-shaped gray matter of the spinal cord contains efferent neural cell bodies and interneurons. There are three important structures within the gray matter:

- The **anterior horn** of the gray matter contains somatomotor neurons.
- The **posterior horn** of the gray matter contains somatosensory neurons.
- The **intermediolateral horn** of the gray matter contains the visceral efferent neurons.

The white matter of the spinal cord primarily contains myelinated axons and glia. It is divided into the anterior, lateral, and posterior columns:

- The anterior column contains the anterior spinothalamic tract, which is responsible for deep touch, and other descending tracts.
- The lateral column contains the descending motor lateral corticospinal tract, which controls ipsilateral limb movement, and the lateral spinothalamic tract, which has fibers that cross through the ventral commissure to the contralateral side of the cord to control pain and temperature sensation.
- The posterior column contains the fasciculus gracilis and fasciculus cuneatus, which are responsible for proprioception, vibration, and fine touch.

The central ependymal canal, located in the middle of the spinal cord, is an extension of the ventricular system and allows the presence of a channel of cerebrospinal fluid (CSF) [2].

Meninges

The meninges are made up of three layers and envelop the spinal cord. The three layers include the pia mater, arachnoid mater, and dura mater. The pia mater is the closest layer to the spinal cord,

1 Cervical Anatomy

the arachnoid mater is the middle layer, and the dura mater is the outermost layer. The denticulate ligaments are located in between exiting spinal nerves and project laterally from the pia to anchor the spinal cord to the arachnoid and dura. These denticulate ligaments provide cushioning and stability for the spinal cord [2, 3].

The epidural space is located in between the dura mater and the vertebrae. The epidural space is bordered anteriorly by the posterior longitudinal ligament (PLL), laterally by the medial aspect of the pedicles and the intervertebral foramina, and posteriorly by anterior aspect of the laminae and the ligamentum flavum. This space contains epidural fat, the internal vertebral plexus, and lymphatics. The CSF, spinal vasculature, and nerve rootlets are located in the subarachnoid space in between the pia and arachnoid mater [3].

Nerve Roots

At each level of the spinal cord, six to eight nerve rootlets exit laterally, become enveloped by the arachnoid and dura mater, and merge to form the dorsal and ventral roots. The ventral motor rootlets exit the spinal cord at the ventrolateral sulcus to form the ventral root, while the dorsolateral sulcus of the spinal cord is where the dorsal sensory rootlets enter. The dorsal root ganglion (DRG) contains the afferent cell bodies and is seen as an enlargement in the dorsal root in the distal aspect of the intervertebral foramen. The nerve roots travel through the intervertebral foramina and, in the cervical spine, pass above the corresponding level of the pedicle. For example, the C7 nerve root exits through the C6 and C7 intervertebral foramen. The exception to this is the C8 nerve root, which passes below the C7 pedicle. The foramen is generally 9–12 mm in height, 4–6 mm in width, and 4–6 mm in length. The nerve roots occupy about one third of the foramen and are located in the inferior half. The superior half contains fat and small veins [2].

The spinal nerve is formed just distal to the DRG, where the ventral and dorsal roots meet. The spinal nerve then divides into the dorsal and ventral primary rami.

The dorsal rami travel posteriorly and divide into motor and sensory branches that supply the muscles and skin of the back of the neck:

- The dorsal ramus of C1 provides motor fibers to the deep muscles of the suboccipital triangle.
- The dorsal ramus of C2 gives rise to the greater occipital nerve.

The ventral rami travel laterally and pass between the scalene muscles to give rise to the following:

- The ventral rami of C1–C4 form the **cervical plexus**, which is located anterolateral to the levator scapulae and middle scalene muscles. The cervical plexus contributes to innervation of the rectus capitis anterior and lateralis, longus capitis and cervicis, levator scapulae, middle scalenes, sternocleidomastoid, and trapezius muscles.
- The ventral rami of C5–T1 form the **brachial plexus**, which provides motor and sensory innervation to the upper extremity [2].

Vagus Nerves

Each vagus nerve exits from the jugular foramen and passes inferiorly within the carotid sheath in between the internal jugular vein and the common carotid artery. The right vagus nerve passes anterior to the subclavian artery and posterior to the brachiocephalic vein, subsequently entering the thorax. The left vagus nerve travels inferiorly between the left common carotid and left subclavian arteries to then enter the thorax.

The recurrent laryngeal nerves arise from the vagus nerves in the inferior part of the neck. The right recurrent laryngeal nerve loops inferior to the right subclavian artery, and the left recurrent laryngeal nerve loops inferior to the arch of the aorta. After looping, the recurrent laryngeal nerves ascend to the posteromedial aspect of the thyroid gland, then ascend in the tracheo-esophageal groove to supply the trachea, esophagus, and all the intrinsic muscles of the larynx except the cricothyroid [2, 6, 7].

Phrenic Nerves

The phrenic nerves arise from the C3, C4, and C5 nerve roots and are formed at the lateral borders of the anterior scalene muscles. They descend under the internal jugular veins and sternocleidomastoid muscles, then pass under the prevertebral layer of the deep cervical fascia, between the subclavian arteries and veins, subsequently traveling to the thorax to supply the diaphragm [2, 6, 7].

Sympathetic Trunks

In the cervical spine, the sympathetic trunks are located anterolateral to the vertebral column and extend superiorly to the level of C1. There are three cervical sympathetic ganglia in the cervical sympathetic trunks, which receive presynaptic fibers from the superior thoracic spinal nerves and their associated white rami communicantes. These cervical sympathetic ganglia then send fibers to the cervical spinal nerves, the thoracic viscera, and the viscera of the head and neck. The three cervical sympathetic ganglia are described as follows:

- The **superior cervical ganglion** is located at the level of C1–C2 vertebrae and is large in size. Postsynaptic fibers from this ganglion form the internal carotid sympathetic plexus, and this ganglion also sends fibers to the external carotid artery and the anterior rami of the superior four cervical nerves.
- The **middle cervical ganglion** is the smallest of the three ganglia and is located on the anterior aspect of the inferior thyroid artery at the level of the C6 vertebra. Postsynaptic fibers from this ganglion travel to the anterior rami of the C5 and C6 spinal nerves, as well as to the heart and thyroid gland. This ganglion is occasionally absent.
- The **inferior cervical ganglion**, in a majority of people, fuses with the first thoracic ganglion to form the cervicothoracic ganglion (**stellate ganglion**). This stellate ganglion is located anterior to the transverse process of C7. Postsynaptic fibers

from this ganglion travel to the anterior rami of the C7 and C8 spinal nerves, the heart, and contribute to a nerve plexus around the vertebral artery [2].

Vasculature

Subclavian Arteries

The subclavian arteries supply the upper extremities and send branches to the neck and brain. The right subclavian artery arises from the brachiocephalic trunk, and the left subclavian artery arises from the arch of the aorta. The branches of the subclavian arteries are important in the blood supply of the neck and include the vertebral arteries, the internal thoracic arteries, the thyrocervical trunks, the costocervical trunks, and the dorsal scapular arteries. The internal thoracic arteries travel inferomedially on both sides into the thorax, and the dorsal scapular arteries supply the levator scapulae, the rhomboids, and the trapezius muscles. The other three branches are described in more detail below [6].

Vertebral Arteries

The major blood supply of the cervical spine comes from the vertebral arteries. One vertebral artery branches off each subclavian artery bilaterally. The vertebral artery typically enters the transverse foramen of the C6 vertebrae and travels superiorly until C1. There, it bends around the lateral mass and posterior arch of C1, travels through the vertebral artery groove and into the foramen magnum where it joins the contralateral vertebral artery to become the basilar artery.

The anterior spinal artery branches off the vertebral arteries at the level of the foramen magnum and supplies the anterior portion of the spinal cord. The posterior columns are supplied by two posterior spinal arteries. The posterior spinal arteries arise from the posterior inferior cerebellar arteries, which are branches of the vertebral arteries. The vertebral arteries and ascending cervical arteries also give rise to segmental medullary arteries; they are typically present at each level to supply the spinal cord, vertebrae, and surrounding tissues [6].

Thyrocervical Trunk

The thyrocervical trunk arises near the medial border of the anterior scalene muscle and has four branches. The largest branch is the inferior thyroid artery, which supplies the larynx, trachea, esophagus, thyroid and parathyroid glands, and the adjacent muscles. Other branches include the ascending cervical arteries, suprascapular arteries, and the cervicodorsal trunk. The terminal branches of the thyrocervical trunk are the inferior thyroid and ascending cervical arteries [6].

Costocervical Trunk

The costocervical trunk arises from the posterior aspect of the second part of the subclavian artery. It divides into the superior intercostal artery, which supplies the first two intercostal spaces, and the deep cervical artery, which supplies the posterior deep cervical muscles.

Veins

The major veins of the neck drain the face, brain, and neck. The internal jugular vein arises as a continuation of the sigmoid sinus and travels out through the jugular foramen. It lies in the carotid sheath with the carotid artery and vagus nerve. It joins with the subclavian vein to form the brachiocephalic vein. The subclavian vein arises as the continuation of the axillary vein at the lateral border of the first rib. It receives only one tributary, which is the external jugular vein. The right and left brachiocephalic veins meet behind the lateral border of the manubrium to form the superior vena cava, which then passes inferiorly to enter the right atrium [4].

Lymphatics

The cervical lymphatic system is responsible for the drainage of tissue fluid, plasma protein, and other cellular debris from the head and neck. The deep lymphatic vessels of the cervical region arise from the deep cervical lymph nodes and converge to form the left and right jugular trunks. The right jugular trunk drains the right upper extremity and right side of the head and neck. It empties into the right lymphatic duct. The left jugular trunk drains into the thoracic duct, which is the larger of the two lymph ducts, which is responsible for draining the rest of the body [4, 6].

Conclusion

In this book, pathological conditions of the neck are discussed. These conditions include cervical strains and sprains, facet-mediated neck pain, discogenic neck pain, cervical radiculopathy, cervical myelopathy, traumatic neck injuries, and rheumatologic causes of neck pain. Having a solid grasp of the normal anatomy of the neck allows for an enhanced understanding of the mechanisms behind the pathologies that will be discussed later in the book.

References

1. Agur, AMR, Dalley AF, Moore KL. (2019). Neck. In Moore's essential clinical anatomy. 6th pp. 595–640). Wolters Kluwer.
2. Dodwad SNM, Khan SN, An HS. Cervical spine anatomy. In: Shen F, Samartzis D, Fessler R, editors. Textbook of the cervical spine. 1st ed. Saunders; 2015. p. 3–21.
3. Ellis H. The anatomy of the epidural space. Anaesth Intensive Care Med. 2009;10(11):533–5.
4. Ellis H. The great veins of the neck. Anaesth Intensive Care Med. 2007;8(1):15–6.
5. Henry J. *Anatomy, head and neck, levator scapulae muscles*, https://www.ncbi.nlm.nih.gov/books/NBK553120/, Accessed 11 Nov, 2021.
6. Moore K. *Moore clinically oriented anatomy*; Ch 7–8.

7. Schuenke M, et al. *THIEME atlas of anatomy: general anatomy and musculoskeletal system*; 85–120.
8. Cuccrullo S. Physical medicine and rehabilitation board review. New York: Demos Medical; 2010.

Cervical Strains and Sprains

Michael Harbus and Leili Shahgholi

Introduction

Cervical axial pain is defined as a pain that is experienced between the inferior occiput and the superior-mid interscapular region, and which localizes to the midline or para-midline regions. Cervical strains are one of the most common disorders of the neck. Cervical strains are musculotendinous injuries that occur because of excessive forces on the cervical spine. 85% of pain that is caused by cervical strain or sprain is the result of acute, repetitive, or chronic neck injuries.

Epidemiology

Neck pain is the fourth leading cause of disability with an annual rate of more than 30% [1]. Distinctive risk factors for neck pain due to strain and sprain include trauma such as traumatic brain

M. Harbus (✉)
Department of Rehabilitation and Human Performance, Icahn School of Medicine at Mount Sinai, New York, NY, USA

L. Shahgholi
Department of Physical Medicine and Rehabilitation, Montefiore Medical Center, Resident, The Bronx, NY, USA

and whiplash injuries and sports injuries (i.e., wrestling, ice hockey, football) [2]. The prevalence of work-related cervical pain is significantly higher in office and computer workers, surgeons, interventionalists, manual laborers, and healthcare workers [3]. Additionally, the prevalence of neck pain is 35–71% among forest and industrial workers. Of note, some studies showed that major workplace factors associated with the condition are low job satisfaction and perceived poor workplace environment [4]. Common factors associated with neck pain include a high body mass index, smoking, a sedentary lifestyle, psychiatric illness, depression, anxiety, poor coping skills, and sleep disorders [5]. There is also a high correlation between neck pain and headache, back pain and arthralgias [4, 5].

Pathophysiology

The cervical spine consists of seven vertebrae, and the related muscles and ligaments which attach to the *skull*, the scapula, *hyoid bone*, *clavicles*, and the *sternum* [6]. The muscles of the neck are uniquely susceptible to muscle strains because cervical neck muscles directly attach to bone via myofascial tissue, whereas muscles in the limbs terminate in tendons prior to attaching to bone [7]. Based on the mechanism of injury, the pathophysiology of cervical strains and sprains differ. For instance, in whiplash injuries, acceleration–deceleration happens post hyperextension (100 ms after a rear-end impact) and followed by 45 degrees of flexion (200–250 ms after impact) [8, 9]. During the event, posterior neck muscles develop eccentric contraction in 90–120 ms, which results in muscle strain and ligamentous sprain. Imaging studies with ultrasound and MRI have shown partial and complete muscle or ligament tear [10]. Deceleration injuries can force anterior longitudinal ligament to merge with the intervertebral disc, which can irritate the disc and provoke pain.

Soft tissue pain disorders with trigger points are another group of common pain disorders in neck area [11]. Although there is controversy about the definition of myofascial pain syndrome, the well accepted term is from pioneers of field Janet Travell and

Simons: a regional pain syndrome in which there is a palpable, discreet nodule within a taut band of skeletal muscle that is spontaneously painful [12]. About 20% of medical consultations due to muscle pain are for myofascial pain syndrome (MPS). Myofascial pain syndrome presents with myofascial trigger points and taut band which can be chronic or active [13]. In the neck area most of the trigger points are in the trapezius, sternocleidomastoid, levator scapula, and rhomboid muscles. Risk factors which predispose patients to myofascial neck pain include muscle imbalance related to cellphone and computer usage [14]. Additionally, obesity may also predispose patients to myofascial neck pain due to the systemic inflammation, structural changes, increased mechanical stress, deconditioned muscles, and psychosocial issues that accompany obesity [4].

Diagnosis

History and Physical

Evaluating for a cervical muscle strain or ligamentous strain requires a thorough and detailed history. Because cervical strains and sprains are often due to muscle overuse, whiplash or "acceleration-deceleration" injuries, or acute trauma, having a patient describe the mechanism of their injury is critical [15]. Mechanisms of injury which commonly lead to cervical soft tissue injury include the following: motor vehicle accidents, sports injury, and work accidents. With any trauma, understanding the direction from which a patient sustained impact is also highly important as rear-impacts are more likely to lead to whiplash injury [16].

Patients should also be asked about lifestyle factors that could contribute to soft tissue injury. Changes in a patient's posture, sleep patterns and position, and work environment can all lead to altered patterns of muscle activation which can then lead to neck pain. When assessing for a soft tissue-mediated neck pain, a history should try to connect a patients neck pain to a specific event, whether it is a trauma or lifestyle change.

On physical examination, patients will demonstrate decreased active and passive range of motion due to muscle guarding. They will also demonstrate tenderness to palpation of their involved muscles and their muscles may be hypertonic on palpation. The most frequently involved cervical strains and sprains are the trapezius and the sternocleidomastoid. When a patient has a cervical strain or sprain without any underlying neurological pathology, they will not present with neurological signs. As such, motor testing, sensory testing, and reflex testing are often normal, and neuroforaminal closing techniques do not elicit radicular pain. Of note, motor examination can occasionally demonstrate give-way weakness due to pain. Additionally, cervical soft tissue pain is often superimposed on an underlying neurological pathology, such as a disc herniation.

Imaging

Imaging is not indicated for cervical strains or sprains unless there is a history of trauma, or neurological findings are present on physical exam. If a history of trauma is given, plain films of the cervical spine with flexion and extension views should be ordered to rule out instability. The most common finding on imaging in cervical strains and sprains is a loss of the cervical lordosis which is due to muscle splinting.

Treatment

Pharmacotherapy

Treatment for cervical strain and sprain is conservative, focusing on controlling a patient's pain and inflammation with the goal of enabling them participate in a functional restoration program. For pain control, the staples of medical management are nonsteroidal anti-inflammatory (NSAID) drugs and acetaminophen. If pain is interfering with a patient's sleep, a short course of muscle relaxants can be beneficial. If patients experience persistent muscle spasm after a cervical sprain or strain, then a course of muscle relaxants can be given.

Among the most commonly used muscle relaxants for cervical myofascial pain are the following medications: cyclobenzaprine, tizanidine, methocarbamol, and baclofen. Cyclobenzaprine is structurally related to the first-generation tricyclic antidepressants, and its site of action is likely the brain-stem, although its exact mechanisms of action is unknown. Tizanidine is an alpha-2 receptor agonist that enhances pre-synaptic inhibition at the spinal motor neurons. Methocarbamol is a centrally acting medication with an exact mechanism that is unknown. Baclofen acts centrally by binding to GABA-B receptors and inhibiting the release of excitatory neurotransmitters [17]. The only muscle relaxant that has strong evidence for cervical spinal pain is cyclobenzaprine. Three randomized trials that investigated using cyclobenzaprine in patients with cervical and lumbar muscle spasm showed that cyclobenzaprine showed clinical efficacy in short-term follow up [10, 18, 19].

Physical Modalities

Physical modalities that can be used to treat cervical strain and sprain include a course of physical therapy, which can incorporate massage, superficial and deep heat, and electrical stimulation and cervicothoracic stabilization exercises. Massage allows for muscular relaxation, the breaking apart of adhesions, vascular changes, and sedation [20]. Both superficial heating and deep heating with ultrasound causes analgesia, muscle relaxation, and increased connective tissue elasticity and also has an anti-inflammatory effect [21]. After a patient has achieved adequate relief of their pain, they can participate in a physical therapy program focusing on cervicothoracic stabilization with the goal of restoring proper biomechanics. This program should be initiated 2–4 weeks after injury. In addition to cervicothoracic stabilization, a physical therapy regimen should include flexibility and range of motion exercises, proprioceptive exercises, and balance exercises [22].

A soft cervical collar can be used early following a cervical strain with the goal of reducing further neck strain. The cervical collar should be worn such that the narrowest side is positioned anteriorly and the widest side is positioned posteriorly. The cervical collar should only be worn for the first 72 h following an injury to prevent the development of soft tissue tightening which can occur with more prolonged use [23].

Conclusion

Cervical strains and sprains are the cause of pain in a significant percentage of patients who present with neck pain [5]. In patients with a suspected cervical strain or sprain, it is essential to have the patients provide a history which includes a detailed report of their mechanism of injury. When examining patients with cervical sprain and strain, the most common findings are limited range of motion due to muscle splinting and guarding due to pain. A thorough neurological exam should also be performed in these patients as muscle spasm often occurs in tandem with discogenic pathology. Treatment for patients with cervical strains and sprains requires pain management with NSAIDs, Tylenol, and, if muscle spasms result from the strain or sprain, muscle relaxants. Physical therapy for patients with cervical strains and strains should involve massage, heat and electrical stimulation for pain relief and cervicothoracic stabilization exercises to allow for restoration of proper movement patterns.

References

1. The prevalence of neck pain in the world population: a systematic critical review of the literature. Eur Spine J. 2006;15:834–48.
2. Bragg KJ, Varacallo M. Cervical sprain. [Updated 2021 Aug 25]. In: StatPearls [Internet]. Treasure Island (FL): StatPearls Publishing; 2021.
3. Epstein S, Sparer EH, Tran BN, et al. Prevalence of work-related musculoskeletal disorders among surgeons and interventionalists: a systematic review and meta-analysis. JAMA Surg. 2018;153(2):e174947. https://doi.org/10.1001/jamasurg.2017.4947.

4. Strine TW, Hootman JM. US national prevalence and correlates of low back and neck pain among adults. Arthritis Rheum. 2007;57:656–65.
5. Cohen SP. Epidemiology, diagnosis, and treatment of neck pain. Mayo Clin Proc. 2015;90(2):284–99. https://doi.org/10.1016/j.mayocp.2014.09.008.
6. Drake RL, Volgl W, Mitchell AW, Gray H. Gray's anatomy for students. 3rd ed. Philadelphia; 2015.
7. Campbell DG, Parsons CM. Referred head pain and its concomitants. J Nerv Ment Dis. 1944;99:544–51.
8. Kaneoka K, Ono L, Inami S, et al. Abnormal segmental motion of the cervical spine during whiplash loading. J Jpn Orthop Assoc. 1997;
9. Tanaka N, Atesok K, Nakanishi K, et al. Pathology and treatment of traumatic cervical spine syndrome: whiplash injury. Adv Orthop. 2018;2018:4765050. Published 2018 Feb 28. https://doi.org/10.1155/2018/4765050.
10. Brown BR, Womble J. Cyclobenzaprine in intractable pain syndromes with muscle spasm. JAMA. 1978;240(11):1151–2.
11. Simons DG, Travell JG. Myofascial pain syndromes. In: Melzack R, editor. Textbook of pain. New York: Churchill Livingstone; 1989.
12. Gerber LH, Shah J, Rosenberger W, et al. Dry needling alters trigger points in the upper trapezius muscle and reduces pain in subjects with chronic myofascial pain. PM R. 2015;7(7):711–8. https://doi.org/10.1016/j.pmrj.2015.01.020.
13. Skootsky SA, Jaeger B, Oye RK. Prevalence of myofascial pain in general internal medicine practice. West J Med. 1989;151(2):157–60.
14. Ye S, Jing Q, Wei C, Lu J. Risk factors of non-specific neck pain and low back pain in computer-using office workers in China: a cross-sectional study. BMJ Open. 2017;7(4):e014914. https://doi.org/10.1136/bmjopen-2016-014914.
15. Cuccurullo S. Physical medicine and rehabilitation board review. New York: Demos Medical; 2010.
16. Braddom RL, Chan L, Harrast MA. Physical medicine and rehabilitation. Philadelphia, PA: Saunders/Elsevier; 2011.
17. Benzon HT, Raja S, Liu SS, Fishman S, Cohen SP. Essentials of pain medicine. 4th ed. Philadelphia, PA: Elseiver; 2018.
18. Bercel N. Cyclobenzaprine in the treatment of skeletal muscle spasm in osteoarthritis of the cervical and lumbar spine. Curr Ther Res. 1977;22:462–8.
19. Basmajian JV. Cyclobenzaprine hydrochloride effect on skeletal muscle spasm in the lumbar region and neck: two double-blind controlled clinical and laboratory studies. Arch Phys Med Rehabil. 1978;59(2):58–63.
20. Wood EC. *Beard's massage: principles and techniques.* 1974.
21. Lehman JF. *Therapeutic heat and cold.* ed 4. 1990.
22. Cole AJ, Farrell JP, Stratton SA. Functional rehabilitation of cervical spine athletic injuries. In: Kibler WB, Herring SA, Press JM, et al., edi-

tors. Functional rehabilitation of sports and musculoskeletal injuries. New York: Aspen; 1998.
23. McKinney LA. Early mobilization of acute sprain of the neck. Br Med J. 1989;299:1006–8.

Facet Joint Pain

Chandni Patel

Introduction

Facet joint syndrome is a condition in which the facet joints of the spine generate pain. The facet joints are paired synovial joints formed from the superior and inferior articular facets of adjacent vertebrae. These joints facilitate flexion and extension motions while limiting rotation and translation of one vertebrae over another. Sensory innervation of the facet joints is provided by the medial branch of the dorsal ramus of the same vertebral level and the vertebrae above. Facet joint syndrome can occur along the cervical, thoracic, or lumbar spinal regions. The focus of this chapter will be cervical facet joint pain.

Epidemiology

The prevalence of reported neck pain varies from 15% to 50% [1]. The incidence of neck pain has been found to increase with age with a peak in middle-aged individuals [2]. A higher prevalence of

C. Patel (✉)
Department of Rehabilitation and Human Performance, Icahn School of Medicine at Mount Sinai, New York, NY, USA
e-mail: chandni.patel@mountsinai.org

neck pain has been found in women [1, 3, 4]. One proposed mechanism for the gender difference can be associated with the fact that cartilage is a sex hormone sensitive tissue [5]. A study by Ha et al. identified the presence of increased estrogen receptor expression in the facet joints of patients with degenerative spondylolisthesis and spinal stenosis [6].

Studies have shown association between neck pain and other disorders including depression, anxiety, smoking, sleep disorders, and sedentary lifestyle. Obesity, in particular, has been shown to be a contributor to musculoskeletal pain due to systemic inflammation, muscle strength decline, and comorbid psychosocial dysfunction [7]. Trauma poses an increased risk for neck pain. Such injuries may follow traumatic brain injury, whiplash, or sports related injuries. Barnsley et al. found 54% of patients with chronic pain after whiplash injury had facet joint syndrome diagnosed by response to facet joint block [8]. Some studies have found an increased prevalence of neck pain among certain occupations. For example, Cote et al. found individual office, computer workers, and manual laborers had the highest incidence of neck pain [2, 9, 10].

Prevalence of facet joint pain varies by spinal level. One study evaluated 500 patients with chronic spine pain. Fifty-five percent of patients with chronic cervical pain were found to have facet joint pain determined by local anesthetic blocks [11].

Anatomy

The facet joints, also known as the zygapophyseal or apophyseal joints, are paired synovial joints composed of a fibrous capsule, articular cartilage, and synovial fluid [12, 13]. Specifically, the articular processes are located between the pedicle and lamina of the vertebrae. The facet joints are formed by the articulation of the superior articular process of the lower vertebrae with the inferior articular process of the upper vertebrae [12, 14]. Except for the C1 and C2 vertebral levels, the paired facet joints and intervertebral discs form the "three joint complex." In the cervical spine, the facet joint surfaces take a convex and concave appearance, respectively [14]. In addition, the surface area of cervical facet joints is about two-thirds the size of the vertebral end plate compared to the smaller surface area of lumbar facet joints [14].

The orientation of facet joints vary by location of the spine relating primarily to the ranges of motion allowed at that region. In the cervical spine, the facet joints are at a 45° inclination from horizontal [11]. The anatomical structure of these joints limit rotation and provide stability in preventing vertebrae slipping while enabling flexion and extension motions [13].

In the cervical spine, the atlanto-occipital and atlanto-axial joints are innervated by the C1 and C2 nerve roots. The C2-C3 facet joint is innervated by the third occipital nerve [15]. Below the C2-C3 facet joint, each facet joint is innervated by the medial branch of the cervical ramus of the corresponding vertebrae and the vertebrae below [15]. For example, the C6-C7 facet joints are innervated by the C6 and C7 medial branches.

Pathophysiology

The most common cause of facet joint syndrome is spondylosis or degeneration of the spine [13]. Degeneration of the spine secondary due to natural wear of the joints is known as osteoarthritis and may be affected by load distribution and alignment [13, 14]. Osteoarthritis of the facet joints will lead to cartilage erosion and inflammation leading to pain. There may be associated ligament hypertrophy or formation of osteophytes [12].

Facet joint degeneration may develop secondary to degeneration of the intervertebral discs. Mechanical loss of disc height and development of segmental instability subsequently increase load on the facet joints leading to cartilage wear [14]. A predisposition of cervical facet joint syndrome has been associated with trauma, inflammatory or rheumatologic disorders, obesity, and spondylolisthesis.

Clinical Presentation

Cervical facet pain often presents with unilateral, non-dermatomal radiating pain to the neck, head, and shoulder [16]. It is dull in character and worse in morning or during periods of inactivity [13]. Less commonly, the pain can be bilateral and radiate to the upper extremities. Patients often present with pain that is intensified by cervical extension or rotation and exacerbated by facet joint palpation or axial loading [13]. If radiating pain is present, other pathology including disc herniations, fractures, and neoplastic causes should be ruled out [13].

Depending on the facet joint level involved, patients will have a certain referral pattern [16].

(a) C1-C2 facet joints: Posterior auricular and occipital region.
(b) C2-C3 facet joints: Forehead and eyes.
(c) C3-C4 facet joints: Suboccipital region and posterolateral neck.
(d) C4-C5 facet joints: Base of neck.
(e) C5-C6 facet joints: Shoulders, interscapular region.
(f) C6-C7 facet joints: Supraspinous and infraspinous fossae.

Physical Examination

A comprehensive physical examination for neck pain involves inspection, palpation, range of motion, strength testing, and special tests of the head, cervical spine, and shoulder.

Inspection

Begin by inspecting the patient's postural alignment. Facing the patient, evaluate for head tilt or rotation, facial asymmetry, and level of the clavicle and acromioclavicular joint. In the lateral view, evaluate for anterior head carriage, curvature of the cervical and thoracic spine, and shoulder rotation. Abnormalities in postural alignment are important to note as it may contribute to increased wear of underlying joint. In each view, evaluate the overlying skin for color changes, rashes, asymmetry, or atrophy which may represent underlying disease.

Palpation

Using palpatory skills, begin by evaluating the skin for temperature changes and sensitivity. Palpate for any effusions or swelling surrounding joints and along the cervical spine, occiput, cervical and upper thoracic paraspinal muscles, trapezius, levator scapulae, and sternocleidomastoid muscles for tenderness. Often, patients with facet-mediated pain will have tenderness to palpation of the cervical paraspinal muscles [12].

Range of Motion

Movement of the cervical spine can be examined through active and passive range of motion. Assessment should begin by having the patient perform neck flexion, extension, side-bending, and rotation. Noting any symmetry or restrictions, the physician should perform passive range of motions to evaluate for any changes in end of the range of motion.

Patients with facet joint syndrome will have decreased cervical range of motion with pain in all ranges of motion but particularly exacerbated by extension and rotation of the neck [16]. Range of motion may be limited in extension and rotation. Range of motion of the shoulder should be evaluated for alternative source of pain.

Neurological Examination

Sensory Testing
Light touch and pin prick sensation should be tested in the cervical dermatomes.

Sensation testing for cervical dermatomes:

(a) C2: 1 cm lateral to the occipital protuberance.
(b) C3: Supraclavicular fossa.
(c) C4: Acromioclavicular joint.
(d) C5: Lateral epicondyle.
(e) C6: Dorsal surface of the proximal thumb.
(f) C7: Dorsal surface of the proximal middle finger.
(g) C8: Dorsal surface of the proximal fifth digit.

Often, there is no sensory impairment in facet joint mediated pain.

Motor Testing

Manual motor testing should be performed to evaluate for weakness in a specific myotome.

Motor testing for cervical myotomes:

(a) C5/C6 nerve root: Deltoid testing with shoulder abduction.
(b) C5/C6 nerve roots: Biceps testing with elbow flexion.
(c) C6/C7 nerve roots: Extensor carpi radialis testing with wrist extension.
(d) C5/C6/C7 nerve roots: Triceps testing with elbow extension.
(e) C8/T1 nerve roots: Abductor digiti minimi testing with finger abduction.
(f) C8/T1 nerve roots: Flexor digitorum profundus testing with distal interphalangeal joint flexion of the middle finger.

Often, there is normal manual muscle testing in facet joint mediated pain.

Reflexes

Testing of upper extremity reflexes can be an important part of the physical exam.

Cervical reflexes:

(a) C5/C6: Biceps.
(b) C5/C6: Brachioradialis.

(c) C6/C7: Pronator teres.
(d) C7/C8: Triceps.

Patients will have normal symmetric reflexes in facet joint mediated pain. If absent or asymmetrical reflexes are present, it may suggest nerve root impingement.

Special Tests

There are two physical examination maneuvers, cervical Kemp's test and spring test, which can be performed to suggest cervical facet pathology.

- Cervical Kemp's Test.
  - Performed with patient in standing or seated position. Induce cervical spine extension with rotation towards side of concern. Reproduction of pain or patient's symptoms is considered a positive test for cervical facet pathology [17].
- Spring Test.
  - Performed with patient in prone position. Examiner applies anterior force over the spinous or transverse processes. Pain or hypo/hypermobility of the joint is positive for facet joint pathology [18].

Diagnosis

A diagnosis of facet joint syndrome begins with a comprehensive history and physical examination. It is also important to obtain laboratory testing and pertinent imaging to rule out other pathology. To facilitate identification of the pain generator, imaging of the cervical spine is often obtained. Although imaging has not been shown to be exceptionally helpful in the diagnosis of facet joint syndrome, initial imaging of plain radiographs of the cervical spine should be obtained to evaluate osseous structures and rule out other pathology. Often, patients will have some abnormality of the facet joints on radiographs. For this reason, physicians may obtain computed tomography (CT) and magnetic resonance imaging (MRI). Imaging may show degenerative changes with joint space narrowing, facet joint hypertrophy and osteophytes suggesting the diagnosis of facet joint syndrome. However, these findings may be present in symptomatic and asymptomatic patients. The gold standard test for facet joint pain is a medial branch block. A positive response to two diagnostic medial branch blocks on two separate events at two or more levels is confirmatory for facet joint mediated pain [13]. One retrospective review followed 500 patients who received diagnostic face joint blocks. A false positive rate of cervical facet joint pain was found in 45% in patients who received a single block [19].

Differential Diagnosis

The differential diagnosis for neck pain is vast. Many disorders may present with symptoms overlapping with facet joint mediated pain and must be ruled out [14, 16, 20].

- Cervicalgia.
- Cervical bursitis.
- Cervical fibromyositis.
- Discogenic pain syndrome.
- Disorders of spinal cord, roots, plexus, and nerves.
- Herniated disc with impingement of the nerve roots.
- Inflammatory arthropathies.
  - Rheumatoid arthritis.
    Of the inflammatory disorders, RA most commonly involves the cervical spine [20]. Rheumatoid arthritis can be associated with cervical spine ligamentous laxity, instability, and subluxation.
  - Seronegative spondyloarthritis.
    Ankylosing spondylitis.
    Reiter's syndrome.
    Psoriatic arthritis.
- Mass or neoplasm of the spine.
- Radiculopathy.
- Spondylosis/spondylolisthesis.

Treatment

Effective management of neck pain due to facet joint syndrome occurs through a multimodal approach. Initial management of a patient with neck pain and suspected cervical facet joint syndrome begins with conservative therapies. Patients begin with physical therapy including heat modalities and lifestyle modifications including weight loss, optimized biomechanics, posture, and workplace ergonomics. Pharmacologic agents including a combination of nonsteroidal anti-inflammatory drugs (NSAIDs) and muscle relaxants may be added to augment pain relief with therapy.

If conservative therapies fail to provide adequate pain relief, patients can undergo injections of the cervical spine including a block of the medial branch of the dorsal ramus or intraarticular injection of the facet joint with anesthetic and steroid. Cervical medial branch blocks commonly performed under fluoroscopic guidance are considered the gold standard for diagnosing facet joint pain. After a medial branch block, patients have been shown to have pain relief for 6 to 12 months [21]. Patients who have had satisfactory relief from two previous medial branch blocks may be considered candidates for radiofrequency ablation of the medial branch nerves which applies heat to the sensory nerve minimizing pain signal transmission [13]. As a final resort, surgery may be considered in patients with spondylolisthesis; however, there are no guidelines supporting arthrodesis for pain relief.

In addition to the primary management of cervical facet joint syndrome, physicians should address coexisting conditions including sleep disturbances, depression, anxiety, and obesity.

Conclusion

Neck pain due to facet joint syndrome can be a progressive, debilitating condition. It is imperative to provide patient education on maintaining a modified lifestyle with physical therapy, medications, and interventional procedures, as appropriate. Interventional procedures including medial branch blocks and radiofrequency ablation are options to manage pain; however, these techniques are not curative and may need to be repeated.

References

1. Binder AI. Neck pain. BMJ Clin Evid. 2008:2008.
2. Gerr F, Marcus M, Ensor C, Kleinbaum D, Cohen S, Edwards A, et al. A prospective study of computer users: I. study design and incidence of musculoskeletal symptoms and disorders. Am J Ind Med [Internet]. 2002;41(4):221–35. https://doi.org/10.1002/ajim.10066.
3. Fejer R, Kyvik KO, Hartvigsen J. The prevalence of neck pain in the world population: a systematic critical review of the literature. Eur Spine J. 2006;15(6):834–48.
4. Cohen SP. Epidemiology, diagnosis, and treatment of neck pain. Mayo Clin Proc [Internet]. 2015;90(2):284–99. https://doi.org/10.1016/j.mayocp.2014.09.008.
5. Rosner IA, Goldberg VM, Moskowitz RW. Estrogens and osteoarthritis. Clin Orthop Relat Res [Internet]. 1986;213:77–83. http://europepmc.org/abstract/MED/2430748
6. Ha K-Y, Chang C-H, Kim K-W, Kim Y-S, Na K-H, Lee J-S. Expression of Estrogen receptor of the Facet joints in degenerative spondylolisthesis. Spine (Phila Pa 1976) [Internet]. 2005;30:5. https://journals.lww.com/spinejournal/Fulltext/2005/03010/Expression_of_Estrogen_Receptor_of_the_Facet.15.aspx
7. Vincent HK, Adams MCB, Vincent KR, Hurley RW. Musculoskeletal pain, fear avoidance behaviors, and functional decline in obesity: potential interventions to manage pain and maintain function. Reg Anesth Pain Med [Internet]. 2013;38(6):481. LP – 491. http://rapm.bmj.com/content/38/6/481.abstract
8. Barnsley L, Lord SM, Wallis BJ, Bogduk N. The prevalence of chronic cervical zygapophysial joint pain after whiplash. Spine (Phila Pa 1976). 1995;20(1):20–5. discussion 26.
9. Hoy DG, Protani M, De R, Buchbinder R. The epidemiology of neck pain. Best Pract Res Clin Rheumatol [Internet]. 2010;24(6):783–92. https://www.sciencedirect.com/science/article/pii/S1521694211000246
10. Côté P, van der Velde G, Cassidy JD, Carroll LJ, Hogg-Johnson S, Holm LW, et al. The burden and determinants of neck pain in workers: results of the bone and joint decade 2000–2010 task force on neck pain and its associated disorders. Spine (Phila Pa 1976) [Internet]. 2008;33(4S) https://journals.lww.com/spinejournal/Fulltext/2008/02151/The_Burden_and_Determinants_of_Neck_Pain_in.11.aspx

11. Manchikanti L, Boswell MV, Singh V, Pampati V, Damron KS, Beyer CD. Prevalence of facet joint pain in chronic spinal pain of cervical, thoracic, and lumbar regions. BMC Musculoskelet Disord [Internet]. 2004;5:15. https://pubmed.ncbi.nlm.nih.gov/15169547
12. Vangindertael J. Facet joint syndrome [Internet]. https://www.physio-pedia.com/index.php?title=Dynamic_Gait_Index&oldid=174683
13. Facet CL. Joint disease [Internet]. 2021. https://www.ncbi.nlm.nih.gov/books/NBK541049/
14. Gellhorn AC, Katz JN, Suri P. Osteoarthritis of the spine: the facet joints. Nat Rev Rheumatol [Internet]. 2012;9(4):216–24. 2013 Apr: https://pubmed.ncbi.nlm.nih.gov/23147891
15. Kim K-H, Kim I-S. Chapter 2—current understanding of spinal pain and the nomenclature of lumbar disc pathology. In: Kim DH, Kim Y-C, Kim K-HBT-MIPST, editors. . New York: W.B. Saunders; 2010. p. 29–45. https://www.sciencedirect.com/science/article/pii/B9780702029134000021.
16. Waldman S. Cervical Facet Syndrome [Internet]. 2019. p. 15, 57–9. https://www-clinicalkey-com.eresources.mssm.edu/service/content/pdf/watermarked/3-s2.0-B9780323547314000153.pdf?locale=en_US&searchIndex=.
17. Stuber K, Lerede C, Kristmanson K, Sajko S, Bruno P. The diagnostic accuracy of the Kemp's test: a systematic review. J Can Chiropr Assoc [Internet]. 2014;58(3):258–67. https://pubmed.ncbi.nlm.nih.gov/25202153
18. Contributors P. Springing Test [Internet]. 2021. p. 1. https://www.physio-pedia.com/index.php?title=Dynamic_Gait_Index&oldid=174683
19. Manchukonda R, Manchikanti KN, Cash KA, Pampati V, Manchikanti L. Facet joint pain in chronic spinal pain: an evaluation of prevalence and false-positive rate of diagnostic blocks. J Spinal Disord Tech. 2007;20(7):539–45.
20. Reiter MF, Boden SD. Inflammatory disorders of the cervical spine. Spine (Phila Pa 1976) [Internet]. 1998;23:24. https://journals.lww.com/spinejournal/Fulltext/1998/12150/Inflammatory_Disorders_of_the_Cervical_Spine.17.aspx
21. Kalichman L, Hunter DJ. Lumbar facet joint osteoarthritis: a review. Semin Arthritis Rheum. 2007;37(2):69–80.

Discogenic Pain

Caroline Varlotta

Introduction

The intervertebral disc (IVD) is one of the main constituents of spine biomechanics. The IVD allows spinal segments freedom and mobility, which enables spinal flexibility. In addition, the IVD provides stability to the spine by dissipating compressive loads and unifying adjacent bony vertebrae into a functional unit. Degenerative changes of mechanical and chemical etiology occur with increasing age and may begin as early as the third decade [1–8]. The etiology is multifactorial and includes demographic risk factors, such as age and gender, along with genetic, environmental, and mechanical factors. In office, physicians may find difficulty differentiating between discogenic neck pain and other etiologies of neck pain. This can be attributed to the varied presentations of discogenic pain—some individuals may find discogenic pain unbearable, while for others it is a benign process. Furthermore, there are no specific pathologic findings on history or physical exam. Imaging may be misleading, as many patients can have degenerative disc findings and with no symptomatology.

C. Varlotta (✉)
Department of Rehabilitation and Human Performance, Icahn School of Medicine at Mount Sinai, New York, NY, USA

This chapter reviews the biomechanics, pathophysiology, presenting signs and symptoms, imaging findings, and treatment of discogenic pain in the cervical spine [9].

Biomechanics/Pathophysiology

The normal adult IVD is an avascular structure between two bony vertebrae. The IVD can be divided into three distinct anatomic substructures—the cartilaginous endplate (EP), the nucleus pulposus (NP), and the annulus fibrosis (AF). The NP located at the core of the IVD is formed from the remnants of the notochord. The amount of water in the disc matrix of the NP is regulated by meshwork of proteoglycans and collagen. The proteoglycans facilitate the binding of water. The increased content of proteoglycans in the IVD allows for it to function as a liquid and dissipate forces. This differs from the AF, a stiff fibrocartilaginous structure composed of type I or type II collagen, oriented in concentric rings. The outer component of the AF densely organized, resulting in increased stability. The AF also has a small amount of elastin to provide elasticity with stretching. The inner AF has a small amount of proteoglycan in addition to its cartilage, lending to slightly higher water content and minimal ability to dissipate forces. The cartilaginous endplate is a thin calcium layer situated on each end of the vertebral body. It allows for diffusion of nutrients into the IVD [10].

There are three clinical and biomechanical stages of spine degeneration described by Kirkaldy-Wallis and Farfan: dysfunction, instability, and stabilization [11]. If one component of the spine's three joint complex is damaged, the effects are experienced by the other two joints in the complex. The most classic example of this concept is disc degeneration—the disc desiccates, providing the initial dysfunction of one component. The result is modified orientation of the superior and inferior facets. Sequelae include inconsistent facet loading, facet hypertrophy, abnormal translation, osteophyte formation, and ligamentous hypertrophy [11–13]. Each of these sequelae are potential pain generators with varying treatments but have vague presentation. To add uncertainty, identification of the presence of disc degeneration on MRI or facet hypertrophy may not be the origin of the patient's pain.

As previously mentioned in this chapter, disc degeneration begins in the NP. In the second decade of life, proliferative chondrocytes replace the residues of notochordal cell aggregates that have been present in the NP since infancy [4]. As the disc continues to age, proteoglycan synthesis decreases and the NP has decreased ability to absorb water, leading to decreased ability to disperse compressive forces. Once the NP becomes dry, granulation tissue appears. In the third decade, the AF begins to replace the fibrous connective tissue network with increasingly hyalinized collagen fibers. Ensuing cellular proliferation death leads to invasion of blood vessels along tears and clefts. General inflammatory pathways are activated as an attempt to repair tears in the AF. As degeneration progresses, other types of collagens may be produced in the AF. The result is a more fibrous and stiff AF unable to handle the compressive forces [13, 14].

Discogenic pain has multiple etiologies. The natural history of degeneration can be affected by comorbidities and prior trauma. Disc space narrowing occurs with increased age and more frequently in women than men, but men are more prone to osteophyte formation [15]. Environmental factors include smoking, obesity, occupational factors. Prior animal studies have demonstrated smokers likely experience impaired blood flow to the disc, leading to decreased synthesis of proteoglycans and collagen [16]. Disc degeneration scores in groups of identical twins discordant for cigarette smoking found smokers had scores 18% higher than nonsmokers [17]. Excessive body weight in obese and overweight individuals was found to lead to a 14-fold greater prevalence of disc degeneration than underweight or normal individuals [18]. This process may begin as early as childhood [19]. Related metabolic disorders, such as diabetes mellitus, can also change the properties of the disc leading to increased prevalence of disc degeneration compared to the general population [20].

The development of disc degeneration depends on nutrient availability as well. The cells of the IVD are very sensitive to extracellular oxygen and pH. As the pH lowers with lactic acidosis from inefficient anaerobic metabolism, proteoglycan synthesis decreases. This decrease in proteoglycans also inhibits the ability of waste products to exit the disc space, contributing to buildup of waste and degeneration. Furthermore, in a healthy individual, nutrients, such as oxygen, will pass through the porous endplate into the disc. If the endplate is impermeable due to calcifications, then nutrients also cannot pass through [13, 21–23].

The genes associated with the development of disc degeneration are categorized into four subtypes. Collagen type I alpha1 gene (COLIA1) is related to disc structure. Certain phenotypes of COLIA1 have been associated with low mineral density, increased bone loss, higher bone turnover, and increased risk of fracture, leading to increased risk of IVD degeneration. Collagen type II alpha2 gene (COL11A2), a gene coding for collagen XI, is also associated with increased risk of IVD degeneration, and subsequent disc bulges and degenerative stenosis. Matrix degrading enzymes have been demonstrated to have a genetic component and can lead to increased risk of disc degeneration. Specifically, IL-1 and IL-6 are associated in the production of inducing enzymes that destroy collagen [19, 24–26].

Aggrecan is a proteoglycan that binds hyaluronic acid, which is another component of the NP that helps to dissipate compressive loads. Polymorphisms of aggrecan may change its properties, resulting in less effective dissipation of compressive loads [27]. MMPs are known to be crucial to the homeostasis of the IVD and matrix turnover. Polymorphisms can lead to increased MMPs and accelerated proteoglycan degradation [28, 29].

Polymorphisms of the gene for the Vitamin-D receptor (VDR) have also been demonstrated to contribute to degenerative disc disease, as VDR plays a significant role in mineralization and remodeling of bones [30, 31]. Other genes, such as SOX9, SPARC, have demonstrated potential to increase risk of disc degeneration, but further research is needed [32, 33].

The inflammatory cascade plays a crucial role in discogenic pain. Degenerated discs have increased amounts of inflammatory mediators [34]. NO and cytokines are produced in the IVD as a response to increased mechanical stress. In patients with disc herniations, there is greater presence of TNF-alpha, IL1B, IL-6 compared to controls. In addition, IL-1, Il-6, NO, MMPs, TNF-alpha,

PGE2, and cytokines are all present in the environment of a degraded IVD [35]. These inflammatory mediators lead to decreased matrix synthesis and increased matrix degradation. The disc will load abnormally due to smaller and fewer proteoglycans limiting the ability to disperse mechanical forces. In this process, there is increased production of waste, which congests the nutrient and waste transport system causing increased cell death and apoptosis. Each of these components contributes to IVD degeneration [33].

Presentation

Cervical discogenic pain can present as acute herniated disc or chronic disc degeneration. In any disc herniation, the patient may present with at level pain because the torn annulus fibrosis has sensory innervation. In addition, an extruded NP can impinge on surrounding neurological structures, causing radiculopathy if the nerve roots are affected and myelopathy if the spinal cord is affected [36]. A detailed motor and sensory exam can identify the level of the lesion [37].

Spondylosis includes degeneration of the disc and may present with vague and overlapping symptomatology, as it is associated with end plate stress, spur and osteophyte formation, and facet arthropathy. Most patients presenting to a physician with degenerative discogenic pain are over 40 years old [37]. The reported symptoms are often poorly localized, such as axial neck pain exacerbated by movement associated with occasional headache. The pain may refer to other areas, such as the shoulder, interscapular zone, or anterior chest wall [38].

Patients presenting with neck pain should always have red flag symptoms ruled out. Pain associated with trauma should be evaluated for fracture and/or instability. If the patient has history of cancer, pain predominantly at night, and/or unexplained weight loss, constitutional symptoms, or failure to improve with reasonable duration of therapy, then consider neoplastic disease. If evidence of systemic inflammatory disease, consider rheumatology referral to evaluate for arthritides. In patients with current or history of intravenous drug use, immunosuppression, or ongoing systematic infection, consider discitis or osteomyelitis. Prior spinal surgery may indicate pseudoarthrosis. Cervical myelopathy should also be referred to a neurosurgeon or orthopedic surgeon [39].

In addition to the general exam questions, the physician may administer the "Neck Disability Index" questionnaire. This investigates 10 areas of activities of daily living with the potential to be affected by neck pain [9, 40].

Imaging

Changes in cervical discs are not uncommon in asymptomatic individuals. One study reported asymptomatic disc degeneration in 86–89% of people over 60 years old [41]. Therefore, imaging should be clinically correlated. Issues exist with imaging in acute cervical disc herniations as well. Boden et al. reported abnormal disc findings in 14% of people who were less than 40 years old, and 28% of people who were older than 40 years. Of these, the disc was degenerated or narrowed at one level or more in 25% of those less than 40 years and almost 60% in those older than 40 years [42].

Spondylosis will have loss of disc height on imaging. CT is superior to MRI in differentiating the contribution of bone hypertrophy to stenosis. However, MRI is superior when assessing for disc bulges and herniations, as surrounding soft tissues can be distinguished from the herniated disc. In addition, mass effect from herniation or bulges on nerve roots and the spinal cord are evident on MRI, whereas they are not usually seen on CT [43]. To evaluate for spondylosis, T2-weighted MRI is most useful, as the normal discs will have intermediate to bright signal. Spondylosis is the most common indication for MRI in the cervical spine. The primary findings will be decreased signal within the cervical discs and focal outpouchings [9]. Whenever reviewing a cervical spine MRI, a physician should also scan for evidence of nerve root or central cord compression [44].

Discography is a diagnostic test involving injection of contrast into an IVD under fluoroscopy. This type of imaging can discern discogenic back pain at specific vertebral levels. During discography, the patient is not sedated and will endorse if the injection pressure at a specific level correlates with his/her pain. The goal of this intervention is to identify specific levels associated with the patient's symptomatology when multiple levels could be involved. As MRI has become more common and spondylosis is identified more frequently, discography has become more common, especially when planning cervical fusion. Discography can also be helpful in patients with prior fusion who have unresolved or recurrent back pain. The true diagnostic value is controversial, as the false positive rate is 10–50% [45–47]. As with MRI, patients with no symptoms may have positive findings on discography. One study demonstrated up to 20% of patients without lower back pain had at least one positive level on discography [48]. This increased to 40% in patients who had history of prior lumbar fusion, but did not have low back pain postoperatively [49, 50] Discography should be reserved for patients undergoing surgical evaluation and planning without clear cut level associated with their symptoms. The risks and discomfort of the procedure do not change management otherwise [51].

Nonoperative Treatment

First-line treatment of cervical discogenic pain without radiculopathy or myelopathy should be treated with physical therapy and medications.

Acetaminophen, or Tylenol, is a weak anti-inflammatory with antipyretic and analgesic effects. Onset is within 30–60 min after ingestion. The incidence of adverse effects is low, and the drug is low cost. Risks include hepatotoxicity in accidental or intentional overdose. It is one of the first-line medications for the treatment of neck pain [52, 53].

NSAIDs are also first line for short-term treatment of neck pain and has the same efficacy as Tylenol [52, 54]. Select COX-2 inhibitors are not more efficacious than nonselective NSAIDs but are associated with lower incidence of gastrointestinal adverse effects [55].

Opioids are not first line due to increased risk of dependence, misuse, abuse, and diversion. Studies have shown opioids have no significant advantage in Tylenol or NSAIDs with regard to symptom relief or return to work [52, 56].

Steroids are potent anti-inflammatory medications that control biosynthesis of prostaglandins and leukotrienes. This class of medications is more advantageous for acute episodes of pain and should be prescribed for 5 days or fewer. The dosing options are Prednisolone 10 mg 3–4 times per day for 5 days or a Medrol dose pack, which is a blister pack titration of methylprednisolone. Diabetic patients should be warned about steroid-induced hyperglycemia [57].

Other medications used for cervical spondylosis and discogenic pain include anticonvulsants, muscle relaxants, tramadol, and tricyclic antidepressants. Anticonvulsants, such as gabapentin and pregabalin, may be indicated for neuropathic pain, as they suppress painful neural activity produced by nerve irritation. Cyclobenzaprine is a muscle relaxant used in patients with associated insomnia. Tizanidine can also be used for muscle spasms associated with back pain but may be more useful in spasticity [57]. Tricyclic antidepressants have conflicting evidence for use and are considered second or third line due to their adverse effects and slow onset [55, 58, 59]. Topical medications, such as Lidoderm patches or diclofenac gel, are not as beneficial for pain secondary to spondylosis.

The use of epidural injections have increased significantly [60]. These injections should be reserved for radicular back pain. Thirty six to forty three percent of patients with spondylosis associated with radiculopathy showed improvement in pain at 1 year evaluations [61, 62].

Gene therapy is also being pursued to promote proteoglycan synthesis in spondylosis. The goal of these treatments would be to increase water content, restore disc height, and its usual properties. In partial thickness tears, gene therapy is limited as the deficit is more commonly in the avascular area where growth factors would not be usually associated with rupture of blood vessels, allowing for the growth factors to have a means to access damaged areas [63]. Further research needs to be completed [64].

Cell therapy is also being studied as a future treatment for degenerative disc disease. Targets of cell therapy would include growth factors, matrix components, such as type II collagen, transcription factors, signal transduction molecules, regulators like SonicHedgehog, anti-inflammatory mediators, inhibitors of apoptosis, and mesenchymal stem cells. The main limitation of this potential treatment is injected growth factors into cells of reduced viability may not be able to restore disc structure once the disc is already damaged. Their presence may also increase metabolic demand, risking further and expedited damage to the disc [65]. Additionally, restoration of the disc may not resolve the patient's symptoms. Further research is needed in this area of treatment as well [64].

Operative Treatment

Chronic degenerative disc changes of spondylosis may resolve spontaneously and usually are treated conservatively [66]. Due to anatomic proximity of the spinal cord and nerve roots to the IVD in the cervical spine, both types of disc herniation (acute and chronic) have potential to result in radiculopathy and myelopathy. Indications for surgery include profound or progressive myelopathy, herniation resulting in severe stenosis, MRI evidence of myelomalacia, progressive radiculopathy, and intractable symptoms that failed conservative management [67]. The primary goal of surgery in these cohorts is to decompress the neural elements to relieve pain, limit neurologic deficit, and improve quality of life [68]. The most optimal functional outcomes occur if the surgical intervention occurs within 6 months of symptom onset [69].

Surgical approach for cervical disc herniation can be both anterior and posterior. Posterior laminectomy and foraminotomy provides direct access to neural elements but limits access to more anterior structures. Currently, anterior discectomy and its variations are the most commonly performed [70].

Cervical total disc replacement (TDR) is indicated for degenerative disc disease at one level between C3 and C7. Cervical TDR allows for direct decompression and removal of the process causing symptoms. Additionally, cervical TDR has higher likelihood of preserving spine biomechanics versus anterior cervical fusion. It also avoids serious complications, such as esophageal injury, dural tear, dysphonia, dysphagia, neurovascular injury, and postoperative airway compromise from edema or hematoma formation [71]. The ideal patient for cervical TDR would have minimal spondylosis, single-level disc herniation, and associated radiculopathy that failed nonoperative management for 6 weeks or has a severe and progressive neurologic deficit. Contraindications for cervical TDR include severe spondylosis, multilevel involvement, bridging osteophytes or ossification of the posterior longitudinal ligament, spondylosis involving C1 or C2, disc height loss of greater than 50%, significant facet joint arthritis, significant spinal deformity, instability, tumor, infection, metabolic bone disease, and morbid obesity [72].

Nucleus pulposus replacement is another potential treatment for mild and moderate degenerative disease [73]. Similar to cervical TDR, NP replacement is best for patients with minimal disruption to other components of the joint, such as the annulus, end plate, and facet joints. The objective is to approximate the physiologic function of the nucleus and protect the integrity of intact components of the joint. The substitute nucleus can be either synthetic replacement or autologous cartilage implantation. Materials used include metals, ceramic, injectable fluid, hydrogels, inflatables, elastic coils. The most commonly used is hydrogels because it functions most similarly to the natural disc [65].

Two other operative alternatives to fusion are interspinous distraction and dynamic stabilization [73]. Interspinous distraction uses a posteriorly placed device to restrict lumbar extension. The result is decreased compression on nerve roots. These implants can be placed under local anesthesia, decreasing risks associated with anesthesia. Another major benefit of interspinous distraction is motion at other levels is spared, reducing postoperative complications, such as pseudoarthrosis, and this method does not contribute to the development of adult spinal deformity [74]. The crucial limitation to note for this approach is an extremity high failure rate demonstrated in one study [75]. Other studies have shown significant complications such as spinal process fracture, device loosening, wing breakage, and dura mater tears [76]. The patient and surgeon should have a conversation regarding risks and benefits to determine if this is the best option.

Dynamic stabilization is the insertion of flexible rods to connect one or more spinal segments. The outcome is stability by altering abnormal loads on the degenerated disc, while avoiding complete fusion. This method allows for controlled movements similar to external braces. It is useful in degenerative disc disease. Risks include loosening at the bone–implant interface, mechanical failure, insufficient stabilization requiring re-instrumentation and fusion, and auto-fusion. One major drawback is the lack of long-term studies and outcomes [12, 77, 78].

Conclusion

Spondylosis and degenerative disc disease may lead to discogenic pain, as the primary function of the IVD is to allow for spinal flexibility and dispersion of mechanical forces. Etiology is multifactorial, and further research is needed to understand, diagnose, and treat discogenic pain. Symptoms are vague and variable but can also be associated with radiculopathy and myelopathy. Additionally, patients with evidence of degenerative changes on imaging may be asymptomatic. Therefore, there is no one treatment for all patients with discogenic pain or spondylosis. Physicians should use physical therapy and medications to lessen symptoms and improve function. Surgical consultation should only be considered in patients with significant radiculopathy, myelopathy, or with intractable pain that failed conservative treatment. Future management may include gene and cell therapy as further research emerges.

References

1. Boos N, Weissbach S, Rohrbach H, Weiler C, Spratt KF, Nerlich AG. Classification of age-related changes in lumbar intervertebral discs. Spine (Phila Pa 1976). 2002; https://doi.org/10.1097/01.brs.0000035304.27153.5b.
2. Ashton-Miller JA, Schmatz C, Schultz AB. Lumbar disc degeneration: correlation with age, sex, and spine level in 600 autopsy specimens. Spine (Phila Pa 1976). 1988; https://doi.org/10.1097/00007632-198802000-00008.
3. Weiler C, Nerlich A, Zipperer J, Bachmeier B, Boos N. SSE award competition in basic science: expression of major matrix metalloproteinases is associated with intervertebral disc degradation and resorption. Eur Spine J. 2002;2002 https://doi.org/10.1007/s00586-002-0472-0.
4. Coventry M. The intervertebral disc: its microscopic anatomy and pathology: part I. anatomy, development and pathology. J Bone Jt Surg. 1945;
5. Coventry MB, Ghormley RK, Kernohan JW. The intervertebral disc: its microscopic anatomy and pathology. J Bone Jt Surg. 1945;
6. Coventry M, Ghormley R, Kernohan J. The intervertebral disc: its microscopic anatomy and pathology: Part III. Pathological changes in the intervertebral disc. *JBJS*. 1945.
7. Siemionow K, An H, Masuda K, Andersson G, Cs-Szabo G. The effects of age, sex, ethnicity, and spinal level on the rate of intervertebral disc degeneration: a review of 1712 intervertebral discs. Spine (Phila Pa 1976). 2011; https://doi.org/10.1097/BRS.0b013e3181f2a177.
8. Berg AJ, Ahmadje U, Jayanna HH, Trégouët P, Sanville P, Kapoor V. The prevalence of lumbar disc degeneration in symptomatic younger patients: a study of MRI scans. J Clin Orthop Trauma. 2020; https://doi.org/10.1016/j.jcot.2020.07.021.
9. Theodore N. Degenerative cervical spondylosis. N Engl J Med. 2020; https://doi.org/10.1056/nejmra2003558.
10. Feng H, Danfelter M, Strömqvist B, Heinegård D. Extracellular matrix in disc degeneration. J Bone Jt Surg Series A. 2006; https://doi.org/10.2106/JBJS.E.01341.
11. Kirkaldy-Willis WH, Farfan HF. Instability of the lumbar spine. Clin Orthop Relat Res. 1982; https://doi.org/10.1097/00003086-198205000-00015.
12. Lee MJ, Lindsey JD, Bransford RJ. Pedicle screw-based posterior dynamic stabilization in the lumbar spine. J Am Acad Orthop Surg. 2010; https://doi.org/10.5435/00124635-201010000-00001.
13. Errico TJ, et al. "Biomechanics of the spine." *Spinal disorders and treatment the NYU-HJD comprehensive textbook*, Jaypee, New Delhi U.a., 2015, pp. 11–17.

14. Sambrook PN, MacGregor AJ, Spector TD. Genetic influences on cervical and lumbar disc degeneration: a magnetic resonance imaging study in twins. Arthritis Rheum. 1999; https://doi.org/10.1002/1529-0131(199902)42:2<366::AID-ANR20>3.0.CO;2-6.
15. De Schepper EIT, Damen J, Van Meurs JBJ, et al. The association between lumbar disc degeneration and low back pain: the influence of age, gender, and individual radiographic features. Spine (Phila Pa 1976). 2010; https://doi.org/10.1097/BRS.0b013e3181aa5b33.
16. Iwahashi M, Matsuzaki H, Tokuhashi Y, Wakabayashi K, Uematsu Y. Mechanism of intervertebral disc degeneration caused by nicotine in rabbits to explicate intervertebral disc disorders caused by smoking. Spine (Phila Pa 1976). 2002; https://doi.org/10.1097/00007632-200207010-00005.
17. Battié MC, Videman T, Gill K, Moneta GB. Smoking and lumbar intervertebral disc degeneration—an MRI study of identical twins. Spine (Phila Pa 1976). 1991;
18. Das UN. Is obesity an inflammatory condition? Nutrition. 2001; https://doi.org/10.1016/S0899-9007(01)00672-4.
19. Samartzis D, Karppinen J, Mok F, Fong DYT, Luk KDK, Cheung KMC. A population-based study of juvenile disc degeneration and its association with overweight and obesity, low back pain, and diminished functional status. J Bone Jt Surg Ser A. 2011; https://doi.org/10.2106/JBJS.I.01568.
20. Park CH, Min KB, Min JY, Kim DH, Seo KM, Kim DK. Strong association of type 2 diabetes with degenerative lumbar spine disorders. Sci Rep. 2021; https://doi.org/10.1038/s41598-021-95626-y.
21. DePalma MJ, Ketchum JM, Saullo T. What is the source of chronic low back pain and does age play a role? Pain Med. 2011; https://doi.org/10.1111/j.1526-4637.2010.01045.x.
22. Kos N, Gradisnik L, Velnar T. A brief review of the degenerative intervertebral disc disease. Med Arch (Sarajevo, Bosnia Herzegovina). 2019; https://doi.org/10.5455/medarh.2019.73.421-424.
23. Kirnaz S, Capadona C, Lintz M, et al. Pathomechanism and biomechanics of degenerative disc disease: features of healthy and degenerated discs. Int J Spine Surg. 2021; https://doi.org/10.14444/8052.
24. Solovieva S, Lohiniva J, Leino-Arjas P, et al. Intervertebral disc degeneration in relation to the COL9A3 and the IL-1β gene polymorphisms. Eur Spine J. 2006; https://doi.org/10.1007/s00586-005-0988-1.
25. Noponen-Hietala N, Virtanen I, Karttunen R, et al. Genetic variations in IL6 associate with intervertebral disc disease characterized by sciatica. Pain. 2005; https://doi.org/10.1016/j.pain.2004.12.015.
26. Noponen-Hietala N, Kyllönen E, Männikkö M, et al. Sequence variations in the collagen IX and XI genes are associated with degenerative lumbar spinal stenosis. Ann Rheum Dis. 2003; https://doi.org/10.1136/ard.2003.008334.

27. Roughley P, Martens D, Rantakokko J, Alini M, Mwale F, Antoniou J. The involvement of aggrecan polymorphism in degeneration of human intervertebral disc and articular cartilage. Eur Cell Mater. 2006; https://doi.org/10.22203/eCM.v011a01.
28. Kalb S, Martirosyan NL, Kalani MYS, Broc GG, Theodore N. Genetics of the degenerated intervertebral disc. World Neurosurg. 2012; https://doi.org/10.1016/j.wneu.2011.07.014.
29. Kawaguchi Y, Osada R, Kanamori M, et al. Association between an aggrecan gene polymorphism and lumbar disc degeneration. Spine (Phila Pa 1976). 1999; https://doi.org/10.1097/00007632-199912010-00006.
30. Videman T, Leppävuori J, Kaprio J, et al. Intragenic polymorphisms of the vitamin D receptor gene associated with intervertebral disc degeneration. Spine (Phila Pa 1976). 1998; https://doi.org/10.1097/00007632-199812010-00002.
31. Videman T, Gibbons LE, Battié MC, et al. The relative roles of intragenic polymorphisms of the vitamin d receptor gene in lumbar spine degeneration and bone density. Spine (Phila Pa 1976). 2001; https://doi.org/10.1097/00007632-200102010-00003.
32. Mayer JE, Iatridis JC, Chan D, Qureshi SA, Gottesman O, Hecht AC. Genetic polymorphisms associated with intervertebral disc degeneration. Spine J. 2013; https://doi.org/10.1016/j.spinee.2013.01.041.
33. Kalichman L, Hunter DJ. The genetics of intervertebral disc degeneration. Associated genes. Jt Bone Spine. 2008; https://doi.org/10.1016/j.jbspin.2007.11.002.
34. Podichetty VK. The aging spine: the role of inflammatory mediators in intervertebral disc degeneration. Cell Mol Biol. 2007; https://doi.org/10.1170/T814.
35. Shamji MF, Setton LA, Jarvis W, et al. Proinflammatory cytokine expression profile in degenerated and herniated human intervertebral disc tissues. Arthritis Rheum. 2010; https://doi.org/10.1002/art.27444.
36. Hunt WE, Miller CA. Management of cervical radiculopathy. Clin Neurosurg. 1986;
37. Errico TJ, et al. "Evaluation and examination of neck pain." *Spinal Disorders and Treatment the NYU-HJD Comprehensive Textbook*, Jaypee, New Delhi U.a., 2015, pp. 36–42.
38. Mechanical disorders of the spine. In: *Low Back and Neck Pain*; 2004. https://doi.org/10.1016/b978-0-7216-9277-7.50018-0.
39. Nordin M, Carragee EJ, Hogg-Johnson S, et al. Assessment of neck pain and its associated disorders. Results of the bone and joint decade 2000-2010 task force on neck pain and its associated disorders. J Manip Physiol Ther. 2009; https://doi.org/10.1016/j.jmpt.2008.11.016.
40. Vernon H, Mior S. The neck disability index: a study of reliability and validity. J Manip Physiol Ther. 1991;

41. Matsumoto M, Fujimura Y, Suzuki N, et al. MRI of cervical intervertebral discs in asymptomatic subjects. J Bone Jt Surg Ser B. 1998; https://doi.org/10.1302/0301-620X.80B1.7929.
42. Boden SD, McCowin PR, Davis DO, Dina TS, Mark AS, Wiesel S. Abnormal magnetic-resonance scans of the cervical spine in asymptomatic subjects. A prospective investigation. J Bone Jt Surg Ser A. 1990; https://doi.org/10.2106/00004623-199072080-00008.
43. Douglas-Akinwande AC, Rydberg J, Shah MV, et al. Accuracy of contrast-enhanced MDCT and MRI for identifying the severity and cause of neural foraminal stenosis in cervical radiculopathy: a prospective study. Am J Roentgenol. 2010; https://doi.org/10.2214/AJR.09.2988.
44. Errico TJ, et al. "MRI of cervical and lumbar spine disorders." *Spinal Disorders and Treatment the NYU-HJD Comprehensive Textbook*, Jaypee, New Delhi U.a., 2015, pp. 102–107.
45. Wolfer LR, Derby R, Lee JE, Lee SH. Systematic review of lumbar provocation discography in asymptomatic subjects with a meta-analysis of false-positive rates. Pain Physician. 2008; https://doi.org/10.36076/ppj.2008/11/513.
46. Carragee EJ, Tanner CM, Yang B, Brito JL, Truong T. False-positive findings on lumbar discography. Spine (Phila Pa 1976). 1999; https://doi.org/10.1097/00007632-199912010-00017.
47. Walsh TR, Weinstein JN, Spratt KF, Lehmann TR, Aprill C, Sayre H. Lumbar discography in normal subjects. A controlled, prospective study. J Bone Jt Surg Ser A. 1990; https://doi.org/10.2106/00004623-199072070-00019.
48. Carragee EJ, Tanner CM, Khurana S, et al. The rates of false-positive lumbar discography in select patients without low back symptoms. Spine (Phila Pa 1976). 2000; https://doi.org/10.1097/00007632-200006010-00009.
49. Carragee EJ, Alamin TF, Miller J, Grafe M. Provocative discography in volunteer subjects with mild persistent low back pain. Spine J. 2002; https://doi.org/10.1016/S1529-9430(01)00152-8.
50. Chelala L, Trent G, Waldrop G, Dagher AP, Reinig JW. Positive predictive values of lumbar spine magnetic resonance imaging findings for provocative discography. J Comput Assist Tomogr. 2019; https://doi.org/10.1097/RCT.0000000000000885.
51. Errico TJ, et al. "Interventional diagnostic procedures: nerve blocks and discography." *Spinal Disorders and Treatment the NYU-HJD Comprehensive Textbook*, Jaypee, New Delhi U.a., 2015, pp.121.
52. Roelofs PDDM, Deyo RA, Koes BW, Scholten RJPM, Van Tulder MW. Nonsteroidal anti-inflammatory drugs for low back pain: an updated cochrane review. Spine (Phila Pa 1976). 2008; https://doi.org/10.1097/BRS.0b013e31817e69d3.

53. Morlion B. Pharmacotherapy of low back pain: targeting nociceptive and neuropathic pain components. Curr Med Res Opin. 2011; https://doi.org/10.1185/03007995.2010.534446.
54. Steinmetz MP, Benzel EC. *Benzel's spine surgery : techniques, complication avoidance, and management Fourth Edition.*; 2016.
55. Salerno SM, Browning R, Jackson JL. The effect of antidepressant treatment on chronic back pain: a meta-analysis. Arch Intern Med. 2002; https://doi.org/10.1001/archinte.162.1.19.
56. Cifuentes M, Webster B, Genevay S, Pransky G. The course of opioid prescribing for a new episode of disabling low back pain: opioid features and dose escalation. Pain. 2010; https://doi.org/10.1016/j.pain.2010.04.012.
57. Errico TJ, et al. "Pharmacologic management of spinal pain: non-narcotics." *Spinal Disorders and Treatment the NYU-HJD Comprehensive Textbook*, Jaypee, New Delhi U.a., 2015, pp. 147–150.
58. Kassis A. Antidepressants to treat nonspecific low back pain. Am Fam Physician. 2008;
59. Savigny P, Watson P, Underwood M. Guidelines—early management of persistent non-specific low back pain: summary of NICE guidance. BMJ. 2009; https://doi.org/10.1136/bmj.b1805.
60. Manchikanti L. Medicare in interventional pain management: a critical analysis. Pain Physician. 2006;
61. Cuckler JM, Bernini PA, Wiesel SW, Booth RE, Rothman RH, Pickens GT. The use of epidural steroids in the treatment of lumbar radicular pain. J Bone Jt Surg Ser A. 1985; https://doi.org/10.2106/00004623-198567010-00009.
62. Buttermann GR. Treatment of lumbar disc herniation: epidural steroid injection compared with discectomy: a prospective, randomized study. J Bone Jt Surg Ser A. 2004; https://doi.org/10.2106/00004623-200404000-00002.
63. Longo UG, Petrillo S, Franceschetti E, Berton A, Maffulli N, Denaro V. Stem cells and gene therapy for cartilage repair. Stem Cells Int. 2012; https://doi.org/10.1155/2012/168385.
64. Errico TJ, et al. "Basic science of degenerative disk disease." *Spinal Disorders and Treatment the NYU-HJD Comprehensive Textbook*, Jaypee, New Delhi U.a., 2015, pp. 3–10.
65. Yue JJ, Bertagnoli R, McAfee PC, An HS. Motion preservation surgery of the spine: advanced techniques and controversies. Am J Neuroradiol. 2009; https://doi.org/10.3174/ajnr.a1707.
66. Zmurko MG, Tannoury TY, Tannoury CA, Anderson DG. Cervical sprains, disc herniations, minor fractures, and other cervical injuries in the athlete. Clin Sports Med. 2003; https://doi.org/10.1016/S0278-5919(03)00003-6.

67. Matz PG, Anderson PA, Holly LT, et al. The natural history of cervical spondylotic myelopathy. J Neurosurg Spine. 2009; https://doi.org/10.3171/2009.1.SPINE08716.
68. Errico TJ, et al. "Operative management of degenerative cervical disorders." *Spinal Disorders and Treatment the NYU-HJD Comprehensive Textbook*, Jaypee, New Delhi U.a., 2015, pp. 324–330.
69. Bertalanffy H, Eggert HR. Clinical long-term results of anterior discectomy without fusion for treatment of cervical radiculopathy and myelopathy—a follow-up of 164 cases. Acta Neurochir. 1988; https://doi.org/10.1007/BF01560567.
70. Decker RC. Surgical treatment and outcomes of cervical radiculopathy. Phys Med Rehabil Clin N Am. 2011; https://doi.org/10.1016/j.pmr.2010.12.001.
71. Pickett GE, Sekhon LHS, Sears WR, Duggal N. Complications with cervical arthroplasty. J Neurosurg Spine. 2006; https://doi.org/10.3171/spi.2006.4.2.98.
72. Errico TJ, et al. "Cervical total disk replacement." *Spinal Disorders and Treatment the NYU-HJD Comprehensive Textbook*, Jaypee, New Delhi U.a., 2015, pp. 347,349.
73. Errico TJ, et al. "Newer motion preservation technologies." *Spinal Disorders and Treatment the NYU-HJD Comprehensive Textbook*, Jaypee, New Delhi U.a., 2015, pp. 332–335.
74. Kondrashov DG, Hannibal M, Hsu KY, Zucherman JF. Interspinous process decompression with the X-STOP device for lumbar spinal stenosis: a 4-year follow-up study. J Spinal Disord Tech. 2006; https://doi.org/10.1097/01.bsd.0000211294.67508.3b.
75. Verhoof OJ, Bron JL, Wapstra FH, Van Royen BJ. High failure rate of the interspinous distraction device (X-Stop) for the treatment of lumbar spinal stenosis caused by degenerative spondylolisthesis. Eur Spine J. 2008; https://doi.org/10.1007/s00586-007-0492-x.
76. Xu C, Ni WF, Tian NF, Hu XQ, Li F, Xu HZ. Complications in degenerative lumbar disease treated with a dynamic interspinous spacer (Coflex). Int Orthop. 2013; https://doi.org/10.1007/s00264-013-2006-2.
77. Bono CM, Kadaba M, Vaccaro AR. Posterior pedicle fixation-based dynamic stabilization devices for the treatment of degenerative diseases of the lumbar spine. J Spinal Disord Tech. 2009; https://doi.org/10.1097/BSD.0b013e31817c6489.
78. Sengupta DK, Herkowitz HN. Pedicle screw-based posterior dynamic stabilization: literature review. Adv Orthop. 2012; https://doi.org/10.1155/2012/424268.

Cervical Radiculopathy

Jonathan Lee, Michael Harbus, and Carley Trentman

Introduction

Cervical radiculopathy is a common disorder that is a manifestation of pain and neurological symptoms due to dysfunction of the nerve root as it exits the cervical spinal cord, most commonly from mechanical compression impingement and/or inflammation. Diagnosis of cervical radiculopathy can be challenging as referred pain from cervical facets, peripheral neuropathies of the upper extremity, and shoulder pathologies can present similarly to cervical radiculopathies. However, the classical presentation of cervical radiculopathy is shoulder and arm pain and/or weakness. Cervical radiculopathies can be treated with conservative measures including therapy, oral medications, and spinal injections, or they can be treated using surgical measures.

J. Lee (✉) · M. Harbus · C. Trentman
Mount Sinai, The Department of Rehabilitation and Human Performance, New York, NY, USA
e-mail: jonathan.lee4@mountsinai.org

Epidemiology

The true incidence and prevalence of cervical radiculopathy is unknown due to the lack of large-scale studies and other associated diagnoses related to the cervical spine. The US military identified 24,742 servicemembers diagnosed with cervical radiculopathy out of 13,813,333 at risk population from 2000 to 2009, an incidence of 1.79 per 1000 person-years [1]. To speak to the possible misdiagnoses or associations with other disorders, a study from Istanbul, Turkey reviewed 220 cases of clinically and radiographically diagnosed as subacromial peripheral impingement syndrome (SIAS) between 2014 and 2016 and found that 35% of patients diagnosed with SIAS also were found to have cervical root compression upon review of the cervical spine MRI on the same side [2]. The US military study identified risk factors of age greater than 40, female sex, White race, and longer service in the military. To contradict, a population-based review of 561 diagnosed patients in Rochester, Minnesota showed greater incidence in men, a male to female ratio of 1.71:1. The most frequently affected nerve root was C7 (~70%) then C6 (~20%) [3].

Anatomy

The cervical nerve root is the branch off the cervical spinal cord that exits the spine through an opening called the intervertebral foramen, representing the beginning of what is commonly referred to as the peripheral nervous system. At each level there are ventral and dorsal nerve roots bilaterally that combine to form the two spinal nerves off each side. At the basics, the spinal nerve carries information both ways, in and out of the spine. The ventral (or anterior) nerve root carries efferent nerves from the spinal cord toward the peripheral nervous system. These are the motor neurons that controls your muscles or preganglionic autonomic neurons. The other dorsal (or posterior) nerve root carries afferent nerves that send sensory information from the peripheral body back to the spinal cord.

5 Cervical Radiculopathy

The cervical spine consists of seven cervical vertebra and eight cervical nerves. Unlike the rest of the spine, the cervical spine is unique that each spinal nerve exits over the corresponding cervical vertebral. For example, the C2 nerve exits between the C1 and C2 vertebra. The C8 nerve exits between the C7 and T1 vertebra.

Mechanism of Injury

The most common mechanism is generally mechanical compression and/or associated inflammation. This can come from a variety of structures and typically differ based on the age of incidence. Typically, younger patients have acute intervertebral disc herniation and older patients have osteophytes. Both however are related to decreased physical space for the nerve to exit the spine through an intervertebral foramen. Other less common causes are post-surgical scar tissue, ligamentum flavum ossification, infection inflammation, and spinal tumors or masses [4]. The mechanism is poorly understood; however, there is an aspect of inflammatory chemical process (via substance P) from the nerve compression that contributes to radicular pain [5].

Clinical Presentation

Based on the anatomy, commonly reported symptoms of cervical radiculopathy range from muscle weakness, pain, numbness, and tingling in the arm. Typically, there are complaints of neck pain due to the sensory innervation of the neck from the dorsal nerve root. Pain patterns can follow the dermatomal patterns, and muscle weakness can follow the myotome pattern.

For example, a 40-year old comes into the office complaining of deep, sharp, radiating pain in the right medial scapula without any prior trauma.

> Patients may or may not have preceding trauma on presentation; however, it should be asked in history taking. Surprisingly there was only a 2% difference in cervical radiculopathy incidence in

MVA patients vs non-MVA patients in cervical radiculopathy [6] and only 14.8% of patients with cervical radiculopathy presented with a preceding trauma or physical exertion in the Minnesota study [3].

Upon physical exam, he is found to have numbness in his lateral forearm and middle finger. He also has mild weakness in elbow extension and decreased reflexes in his right triceps tendon. This is a classical presentation since:

- The pain the medial scapula is hypothesized to be due to the C7 nerve root dorsal rami that are found to end in the semispinalis cervicis or capitis muscles [7].
- The numbness typically follows the dermatome pattern of C7 to the middle finger and posterior forearm.
- The weakness follows the myotome pattern of C7 to the triceps.
- The diminished reflex follows the reflex arm mediated by the C6 and C7 nerve roots.

Diagnosis

Although the weakness typically presents based on associated myotomes and sensory pain is related to respective dermatomes of each nerve root level, symptoms may vary due to if multiple nerve roots are involved, the overlapping of adjacent dermatome innervations, and contributions of multiple myotomes by one nerve root. A small study with 169 patients found that pain reported by cervical radiculopathy patients was non-dermatomal in 69.7% of cases [8]. This could also be due to anatomical differences in patients.

There are physical exam prevocational tests to help diagnose radiculopathy, however are poor at ruling it out.

- The Spurling test, which tests the provocation of pain by extending the head and rotating toward the side of pain and applying light axial compression from the head, is based on the

idea of narrowing the intervertebral foramen the spinal nerve is running through. This test was found to have high specificity however low sensitivity.
- The neck distracting test, which tests for relief of pain when applying light traction from the head, is based on the idea of opening the intervertebral foramen for the spinal nerve. This test was also found to have a high specificity and low sensitivity [9].

Radiologically, MRI is the image of choice if physical exam and history includes radiculopathy high in the differential. The superior images of soft tissue make MRI superior than CT and X-rays in helping to diagnose radiculopathy. Cervical X-rays are helpful to see the degree of cervical spondylosis that predisposes older patients to radiculopathy; however, it is not enough to diagnose alone. In addition, it is important to understand that if there is radiological evidence of foraminal stenosis or disc herniation, clinically the patient may be asymptomatic. Vice versa a patient may be symptomatic despite minimal findings on MRI. An MRI study of 78 patients with radiculopathy symptoms had two neuroradiologists review MRI images while blinded to clinical information. About 73% of the clinically affected root was found reported as compressed on MRI; however, 45% of MRIs showed root compression that did not correlate to clinically affected roots, and 13–15% of cases were read as normal MRIs. Without clinical correlation, even superior MRI images showed high levels of false positives and false negatives [10].

If MRI findings and physical exam finds do not fully correlate, the next step would be electrodiagnostic studies (electromyography and nerve conduction testing) to help differentiate a cervical radiculopathy from peripheral impingement syndromes. A clinical pearl is to not proceed with the EMG/NCS too early after onset as the sharp wave potentials and fibrillations potentials seen on testing may not appear until up to 3 weeks after onset [11].

All these factors only further show that physical exam findings, patient complaints, and radiological evidence should be combined to produce as accurate diagnoses as possible.

Management

Treatment is largely nonoperative conservative first-line treatment with surgery reserved for severe cases. Physical therapy is largely the beginning step for treatment including range of motion exercises, soft tissue mobilization, cervical neck traction, and modalities of ice, heat, and electrical stimulation. To help augment improvement in therapy, pain management is helpful with NSAIDs and acetaminophen, especially to help decrease inflammation contributions. For more severe pain, there is a role for short-term opioids, short-term steroids, or gabapentin for neuropathic pain; however, all these modalities will not cure the pain. Conservative treatment is largely not supported by high-quality evidence and mostly an aspect of anecdotal evidence [12]. The management should largely be patient-based individualized plan based on risks and comorbidities. NSAIDs use can be limited to kidney disease and steroids can complicate diabetes management and cause mood effects. Acupuncture may also be a low-risk modality to help with pain.

After failure of these treatments, the next discussed option may be an epidural steroid injection into the suspected nerve root level. This approach will place a direct steroid and/or lidocaine mixture into the affected nerve root space to provide short-term pain relief and decrease the inflammatory process. Multiple studies have shown that epidural steroid injections have short-term pain relief of 50% relief for at least 4 weeks after injection. These effects are typically not seen long term. The conversation around injections are that the goal of these injections is not to cure the pain, like oral medications, but to help alleviate pain to augment subsequent physical therapy and exercises [13, 14]. Studies have not been done to compare epidural injections with and without subsequent physical therapy to evaluate for long-term benefits. Again, the management is largely patient dependent on functional needs as any injection/medication/surgery has associated risks and side effects.

Failure of conservative treatment, including epidural injections, or significant severe symptoms of nerve damage are indications for surgical referral. Surgical options are anterior cervical decompression and fusion, cervical disk arthroplasty, and posterior foraminotomy [12]. The idea behind these operations are to open the space that is compressing the nerve root, and, if needed, adding a fusion component if spinal stabilization is necessary. In patients undergoing conservative treatment with worsening symptoms, surgery may not recover neurologic function; however, it may stop further deterioration.

Outcomes

Most patients do well with appropriate treatment. The difficulty in managing is due to no clear guidelines with superior outcomes. A meta-analysis looking at outcomes of cervical radiculopathy showed that most patients presented with intense pain and moderate levels of disability but had a time to complete recovery range of 24–36 months in ~83% of patients. The most significant improvements occurred within 4–6 months of onset. Interestingly this study also found that workers' compensation claims had a poorer prognosis and also involved more invasive treatments of epidural injections and surgery [15]. In the Minnesota study, 31.7% had reoccurrence and 26% underwent surgery. At final follow-up, 90% of patients have resolved symptoms or mild symptoms. In a multicenter study of 246 patients with cervical radiculopathy, 51 (33%) of the available 155 patients with follow-up underwent surgery [16]. In a small study with 26 patients, 24 were treated without surgery and 21 returned to the same job with 1 retiring [17].

Conclusion

Cervical radiculopathies result from any structural change that results in compression of a cervical nerve root as it exits through the neuroforamen. Cervical radiculopathies present as neck pain that radiates down the arm; however, they do not regularly follow a dermatomal pattern, as is often taught. Diagnosis requires a thorough physical exam and MRI and EMG/NCS can both provide useful information in confirming the diagnosis of cervical radiculopathy if the MRI or EMG/NCS findings correlate with a patients symptomatology. Patients with cervical radiculopathy may try either noninterventional or interventional strategies to ameliorate their symptoms, with interventions being reserved for patients with functional limitations or neurological deficits.

References

1. Schoenfeld AJ, George AA, Bader JO, Caram PM. Incidence and epidemiology of cervical radiculopathy in the United States military: 2000 to 2009. J Spinal Disord Tech. 2012;25(1):17–22.
2. Dernek B, Aydoğmuş S, Duymuş TM, et al. The incidence of impingement syndrome in cases of cervical radiculopathy: an analysis of 220 cases. J Back Musculoskelet Rehabil. 2020;33(3):363–6.
3. Radhakrishnan K, Litchy WJ, O'Fallon WM, Kurland LT. Epidemiology of cervical radiculopathy. A population-based study from Rochester, Minnesota, 1976 through 1990. Brain. 1994;117(Pt 2):325–35.
4. Song JY, Park JH, Roh SW. Ossified ligamentum flavum causing cervical myelopathy. Korean J Spine. 2012;9(1):24–7.
5. Cornefjord M, Olmarker K, Farley DB, Weinstein JN, Rydevik B. Neuropeptide changes in compressed spinal nerve roots. Spine (Phila Pa 1976). 1995;20(6):670–3.
6. Braddom RL, Spitz L, Rivner MH. Frequency of radiculopathies in motor vehicle accidents. Muscle Nerve. 2009;39(4):545–7.
7. Mizutamari M, Sei A, Tokiyoshi A, et al. Corresponding scapular pain with the nerve root involved in cervical radiculopathy. J Orthop Surg (Hong Kong). 2010;18(3):356–60.
8. Murphy DR, Hurwitz EL, Gerrard JK, Clary R. Pain patterns and descriptions in patients with radicular pain: does the pain necessarily follow a specific dermatome? Chiropr Osteopat. 2009;17:9.
9. Rubinstein SM, Pool JJ, Tulder M van, Riphagen II, de Vet H. *A systematic review of the diagnostic accuracy of provocative tests of the neck for diagnosing cervical radiculopathy*. Centre for Reviews and Dissemination (UK); 2007.
10. Kuijper B, Tans JTJ, van der Kallen BF, Nollet F, Lycklama A, Nijeholt GJ, de Visser M. Root compression on MRI compared with clinical findings in patients with recent onset cervical radiculopathy. J Neurol Neurosurg Psychiatry. 2011;82(5):561–3.
11. Han JJ, Kraft GH. Electrodiagnosis of neck pain. Phys Med Rehabil Clin N Am. 2003;14(3):549–67.

12. Corey DL, Comeau D. Cervical radiculopathy. Med Clin North Am. 2014;98(4):791–9. xii
13. Woods BI, Hilibrand AS. Cervical radiculopathy: epidemiology, etiology, diagnosis, and treatment. J Spinal Disord Tech. 2015;28(5):E251–9.
14. Engel A, King W, MacVicar J. Standards division of the international spine intervention society. The effectiveness and risks of fluoroscopically guided cervical transforaminal injections of steroids: a systematic review with comprehensive analysis of the published data. Pain Med. 2014;15(3):386–402.
15. Wong JJ, Côté P, Quesnele JJ, Stern PJ, Mior SA. The course and prognostic factors of symptomatic cervical disc herniation with radiculopathy: a systematic review of the literature. Spine J. 2014;14(8):1781–9.
16. Sampath P, Bendebba M, Davis JD, Ducker T. Outcome in patients with cervical radiculopathy. Prospective, multicenter study with independent clinical review. Spine (Phila Pa 1976). 1999;24(6):591–7.
17. Saal JS, Saal JA, Yurth EF. Nonoperative management of herniated cervical intervertebral disc with radiculopathy. Spine (Phila Pa 1976). 1996;21(16):1877–83.

Cervical Myelopathy

Toqa Afifi, Karolina Zektser, and Aditya Raghunandan

Introduction

Cervical myelopathy, or symptomatic spinal cord compression [1], is defined as spinal cord dysfunction of insidious onset, more commonly diagnosed in the elderly and is caused by compression of the cervical spinal cord [2]. Compression of the cervical spinal cord results in neurological deficits that vary in presentation depending on the level of compression, etiology and mechanism of compression, and age and severity of the disease. Commonly reported symptoms include neck pain or stiffness, numbness, paresthesia, ataxic gait, and weakness in the upper and lower extremities and in later stages of the disease may present with additional bowel and bladder dysfunction [2–5].

T. Afifi (✉) · K. Zektser
Physical Medicine and Rehabilitation Residency Program, Spaulding Rehabilitation Hospital - Harvard Medical School, Charlestown, MA, USA
e-mail: tafifi@mgh.harvard.edu; kzektser@northwell.edu

A. Raghunandan
Spine and Sports Medicine, Department of Rehabilitation Medicine, Long School of Medicine at the University of Texas Health Science Center at San Antonio, San Antonio, TX, USA
e-mail: raghunandan@uthscsa.edu

© The Author(s), under exclusive license to Springer Nature Switzerland AG 2022
M. Harbus et al. (eds.), *A Case-Based Approach to Neck Pain*, https://doi.org/10.1007/978-3-031-17308-0_6

"Degenerative Cervical Myelopathy"(DCM) is a term coined in 2015 to describe the nontraumatic, degenerative causes of cervical myelopathy that result in structural and functional abnormalities in the spinal cord through static and dynamic factors. It includes spondylosis, disc herniation, facet arthrosis, ligamentous hypertrophy, calcification, and ossification [5–7].The cervical column is particularly vulnerable to degenerative changes due to its mobility and these changes are more commonly seen with increasing age [4].

Cervical myelopathy is a disorder that encompasses multiple neurological conditions and can be categorized into extrinsic and intrinsic neural etiologies. Before discussing the different etiologies, it is important to clarify some nomenclature. In certain books and literature, "**cervical spinal stenosis**" is synonymously used with "cervical myelopathy". However, while cervical myelopathy refers to the compression of the spinal cord, cervical spinal stenosis refers to the pathological (or congenital) narrowing of the spinal canal. Pathological narrowing of the spinal canal may cause compression of the spinal cord and potentially to symptomatic compression (cervical myelopathy). Cervical spinal stenosis can be congenital or acquired. Congenital stenosis could be structural secondary to short pedicles or in association with developmental disorders such as achondroplasia, trisomy 21, and others. Acquired cervical spinal stenosis is most commonly due to degenerative, hypertrophic or age-related changes but could also be due to other conditions such as ossification of the posterior longitudinal ligament (OPLL), atlantoaxial subluxation in rheumatoid arthritis or degenerative spondylolisthesis [1].

Myelomalacia

Myelomalacia has traditionally been defined as a radiographic finding on magnetic resonance imaging (MRI) visualized as a poorly defined region of spinal cord signal that appears hypointense on T1 and hyperintense on T2 weighted sequences [8]. Patients with cervical spondylotic myelopathy (CSM) can also demonstrate myelomalacia with the same characteristic MRI signal intensities [9]. Clinical correlation and prognostic factors utilizing these imaging findings, however, are more nuanced and not as clear. Increased signal intensity (SI) in T2 sequences can be classified into two grades, type 1 and type 2 [10, 11]. Type 1 or "faint, fuzzy, indistinct borders" 'correlate closely to reversible changes, while type 2 or "intense, well-defined borders" correlate with irreversible histological damage. These classifications were based on a histopathologic spinal cord study that showed severe changes (microcavitation, spongiform changes, and necrosis) have a higher water content, resulting in more intense borders. However, milder histological changes, such as edema, demyelination, and Wallerian degeneration, produce less well-defined borders. Both studies demonstrated improvements in SI in type 1 postsurgically, confirming that milder signal changes are reversible [10, 11]. A systematic review by Tetreault et al. provides a weak recommendation for using combined T1/T2 signal change, SI ratio, and a greater number of SI segments on a T2WI for post-surgical prognosis, as they were found to be negatively associated with outcome. Unfortunately, there currently are no reliable standardized classification methods to quantify the degree of signal change [12].

Etiologies

Various etiologies can lead to the symptomatic compression of the spinal cord (Table 6.1). Causes of cervical myelopathy can be divided into extrinsic and intrinsic neural etiologies. Extrinsic neural etiologies are conditions that are external to the spinal cord and cause mechanical compression of the cord, potentially leading to myelopathy. Intrinsic neural etiologies are primary pathologies that occur within the spinal cord itself causing the symptoms of myelopathy. The clinical significance of this categorization comes from intrinsic pathologies being used as a differential for mechanically compressive myelopathy etiologies.

Risk Factors

There are certain hereditary factors that have been shown to be correlated with the development of degenerative cervical myelopathy. Literature has shown MMP-2 and collagen IX genes to be

Table 6.1 Categorization of the etiologies of cervical myelopathy based on extrinsic (due to external mechanical compression of the cord) and intrinsic (due to diseases of the cord itself) - Adapted from Interventional Spine, Chapter 50 and Nouri A, et al.; 2015 [2, 6]

Etiologies of Cervical Myelopathy [2]			
	Extrinsic		Intrinsic
Pathophysiology	Pathologies of the structures surrounding the spinal cord contribute to the mechanical compression of the cord		Primary pathology is in the spinal cord itself
Types	Degenerative Cervical Myelopathy	Cervical Spondylosis	Viral Infections
		Cervical Disc Herniation	Neoplasms
		Ossification of the Posterior Longitudinal Ligament	Vascular Diseases
		Calcification of the Ligamentum Flavum	Motor Neuron Disease (e.g.: ALS)
		Rheumatoid Arthritis	Multiple Sclerosis
		Spinal Tumors	Radiation Myelopathy
		Epidural Abscess	Nutritional Myelopathy
		Destructive Spondyloarthropathy	Syringomyelia

associated with degenerative disc disease and collagen VI and XI to be associated with ossification of the posterior longitudinal ligament [6].

Degenerative changes of the bone, ligaments, and intervertebral discs cause a disruption of cervical kinetics. Patients with certain movement disorders such as Parkinson's, cerebral palsy, and other neurodegenerative diseases of the cortical or basal ganglia may also develop progressive myelopathy due to dyskinesia and dystonia. Skeletal dysplasias, torticollis, Tourette syndrome, and psychogenic diseases may also increase the risk of degeneration due to static and dynamic injury mechanisms.

Certain medical conditions increase the risk of cervical degeneration. Patients who have hypoparathyroidism, poly-hypophosphatemic rickets, and short sleeping hours are also at increased risk of developing OPLL. Non-insulin dependent diabetes mellitus increases the general ossification of spinal ligaments. Individuals predisposed to atlantoaxial subluxation because of Rheumatoid Arthritis or Trisomy 21 also face an increased risk. Congenital stenosis is prevalent in disorders such as achondroplasia, Klippel-Feil syndrome, and Morquio syndrome [1].

Environmental factors, such as tobacco, use also increases the risk since smoking decreases bone mineral density, increases fracture risk as well as increases the incidence rates of degenerative disc disease [6]. Trauma, occupations requiring weight bearing on the head, tumors, metastatic disease, and abscess formation also increase the risk of cervical degeneration.

Demographics

Any demographic of patients with increased risk factors for cervical spine canal narrowing are more predisposed to compression of the cervical cord and, therefore, cervical myelopathy.

Cervical myelopathy is the most common cause of spinal cord impairment in the elderly population. It is also the most common form of spinal cord injury in adults and makes up 54% of nontraumatic spinal cord injury in North America [13–15].

With age, many degenerative and hypertrophic changes progressively occur in the intervertebral discs, facet joints, ligamentum flavum, and uncovertebral joints (Joints of Luschka) that cause neural foraminal narrowing and thereby impinge the cervical spinal cord. Other degenerative changes such as spondylolisthesis, spondylosis, osteophytes, disc herniations, disc calcifications, and facet hypertrophy result in biomechanical changes that also obstruct the vertebral canal resulting in cervical myelopathy. These degenerative changes are present in 75%–85% of the population by the age of 65 [1]. Males present with a higher incidence of canal stenosis from spondylosis at a ratio of 3:2 and more severe stenosis at the primary level of pathology which later can develop into myelopathy [16].

Cervical myelopathy can overlap with many other neurological conditions and is often underdiagnosed [6]. The incidence and prevalence of degenerative cervical myelopathy is about 41 and 605 per million in North America. The incidence of hospitalizations due to cervical spondylotic myelopathy is 4.04/100,000 leading to an increase in surgical rates [6]. About 1.6 per 100,000 inhabitants underwent surgical intervention for cervical myelopathy [17, 18].

The Asian population is more predisposed to the ossification of the posterior longitudinal ligament and ligamenta flava and therefore are at a higher risk of developing myelopathy [19].

Degenerative Cervical Myelopathy

Degenerative Cervical Myelopathy (DCM) refers to nontraumatic, degenerative causes of cervical myelopathy that result in structural and functional abnormalities in the spinal cord through static and dynamic factors. It includes spondylosis, disc herniation, facet arthrosis, ligamentous hypertrophy, calcification, and ossification [5–7]. The cervical column is particularly vulnerable to degenerative changes due to its mobility and these changes are more commonly seen with increasing age [4].

DCM is more commonly diagnosed in the elderly above the age of 50, in men more than women with a 3:1 male to female ratio of patients [3]. Exact incidence of DCM is difficult to determine for multiple reasons:

- Differences in terminology:
    The term "Degenerative Cervical Myelopathy" was introduced in 2015 and was previously diagnosed depending on its etiology which caused much ambiguity when referring to this collective set of diseases.
- Many patients go undiagnosed:
    A small study showed 18% of 66 patients with hip fractures were found to have undiagnosed cervical myelopathy [18]. DCM diagnosis could be missed because:

1. Early clinical features may be subtle and overlap with other neurological conditions [16].
2. Incomplete neurological assessments performed by physicians [17].
3. Lack of awareness of the disease.
- Radiological findings can be present in asymptomatic patients:
    If you randomly select people between the ages 40 and 80, around 59% of them will have incidental cervical cord compression detected on MRI [20]. 8% of these patients will develop DCM after 1 year and around 22% in total will develop DCM later in life [21].

Cervical Spondylotic Myelopathy

Cervical spondylotic myelopathy (CSM) is the most common cause of compressive cervical myelopathy [2]. Cervical spondylosis is the degeneration of the intervertebral discs of the cervical spine that develop spontaneously with age, repetitive daily use, occasional trauma, and excessive use, with nutritional or environmental factors, or with a combination of these factors. As the intervertebral disc degenerates, a cascade of altered weight-bearing biomechanics causes uneven pressure placement on the vertebra resulting in adaptive remodeling of the spine through osteophyte formation or "spurs." Chronically, this pathologic process may be further complicated by acute disc herniation. The bulging of the annulus fibrosus is referred to as "soft" disc herniation. In cervical spondylosis, the enlarging calcification of a posterior marginal osteophyte is referred to as a "hard" disc herniation and may co-occur with a soft disc herniation [6, 22].

Cervical spondylosis as a degenerative process is a common finding in the asymptomatic elderly and is of no clinical concern unless it correlates with corresponding neurological symptoms on history and physical exam. Depending on where the osteophytic remodeling and "hard" herniation occurs (to the side and towards the nerve root or posteriorly towards the spinal cord itself), a specific neurological symptomatology will develop. Radiculopathy occurs when the nerve root is impinged resulting in neurological deficits corresponding to that specific nerve root. Cervical spondylotic myelopathy occurs when spondylosis results in narrowing of the vertebral foramen with the compression of the spinal cord.

It is easily differentiated from radiculopathy as cervical spinal cord damage will result in neurological deficits observed in all four extremities [6, 16, 22].

Cervical Disc Herniation

Cervical Disc Herniation (CDH) refers to isolated "soft" disc herniation. As previously mentioned, "soft" disc herniation is the bulging of the intervertebral disc while "hard" disc herniation is the posterior enlargement of osteophytic spurs into the spinal canal. Posterolateral herniations cause nerve root impingement and result in radiculopathy while posteromedial herniations that bulge centrally and compress the spinal cord result in cervical myelopathy [2, 22].

Soft disc herniation can be an isolated etiology for cervical myelopathy in severe cases of disc degeneration that causes significant bulging of the intervertebral disc into the spinal cord. However, soft disc herniations more commonly present as mild cases of disc bulging accompanied by progressive degenerative and osteophytic changes leading to superimposed "hard" disc herniations presenting in the elderly as cervical spondylotic myelopathy [2, 22, 23].

Given their interrelated pathophysiologies, CSM and CDH are sometimes grouped together under the term **"Degenerative Disc Disease" (DDD)** as one of the osteoarthritic etiologies of DCM.

Isolated soft disc herniations causing cervical myelopathy are more commonly seen in younger patients with a history of cervical spinal trauma being a common predisposing factor [24]. The clinical presentation of cervical myelopathy in the setting of isolated soft disc herniation would be more acute with rapidly progressing neurological deficits compared to cervical myelopathy in soft with superimposed hard disc herniations. The latter mixed pathophysiology would more likely present as a CSM clinical picture [6, 23].

Ossification of the Posterior Longitudinal Ligament

The posterior longitudinal ligament (PLL) is a paravertebral ligament that originates from the dorsum of C2 vertebra and courses distally towards the sacrum and functions to resist hyperflexion and distraction [25, 26]. The **Ossification of the Posterior**

Longitudinal Ligament (OPLL) accounts for approximately 10% of cervical myelopathy patients [27] and is defined as a hyperostotic pathologic process of the PLL of uncertain pathophysiology that results in the replacement of the PLL's ligamentous tissue with lamellar bone [2, 25, 27].

OPLL is more commonly diagnosed in men (2:1 male to female ratio) and in older individuals (ages 40–60) [28]. OPLL is traditionally known to be a disease associated with the Japanese and other East Asian populations; however, more recent research is challenging this long held view of the disease epidemiology. Recent data has shown the sporadic distribution of the disease and the prevalence across various ethnicities [29–32]. The overall prevalence of cervical OPLL has been found to be consistently around 1.9–2.5%. OPLL has been found in 1.9–4.3% of the Japanese, 0.8–3% of Southeast Asian, and 0.01–1.7% in North American and European populations [29, 31, 33–35]. A cross-sectional study in 2015, San Francisco of 3161 patients revealed prevalence of 1.3% in Caucasian Americans, 4.8% in Asian Americans, 1.9% in Hispanic Americans, 2.1% in African Americans, and 3.2% in Native Americans [32].

Cervical OPLL is more common than thoracic OPPL and presents with a variable neurological sequelae of myelopathy and radiculopathy depending on the affected structures [33, 36]. Primary (idiopathic) OPLL has shown to be associated primarily with Diffuse Idiopathic Skeletal Hyperostosis (DISH) and Ossification of the Ligamentum Flavum but also with other comorbidities and factors such as diabetes mellitus, obesity, vitamin A rich diet, exercise, and mechanical stress to the head. Secondary OPLL is associated with hypophosphatemic rickets and endocrine disorders such as hypoparathyroidism and acromegaly. OPLL has also been linked to multiple genes including BMP2, BMP4, COL6A1, COL11A2, NPPS, and TGFβ [25, 33].

OPLL has been classified into four types based on morphology:

- Localized: Ossification confined to the disc space.
- Segmental: Ossification is fragmented posterior to the vertebral body throughout the cervical spine.

- Continuous: Ossification extends across multiple consecutive vertebra.
- Mixed: Combination of segmental and continuous picture of ossification [37].

Ossification and Calcification of the Ligamentum Flavum

Limited research has been done on **Calcification of the Ligamentum Flavum (CLF).** CLF is known to occur more commonly in females and is associated with pseudogout (calcium pyrophosphate dihydrate deposition disease) [6, 38]. It is also potentially associated with hypercalcemia, hyperparathyroidism, hemochromatosis, and renal failure. CLF more commonly affects the cervical spine as compared to **Ossification of the Ligamentum Flavum (OLF)** which affects the thoracic spine and also differs from CLF in histopathology. OLF is a metaplastic process more common in older men with similar pathology to OPLL in that it results in lamellar bone formation from endochondral ossification that bridges the upper and lower edges of two adjacent laminae. OPLL and OLF have differing natural histories; however, they share similar pathologies which could possibly be attributed to common associations with certain genetic variants and mutations such as in NPPS, COL6A1, and RUNX2 [6]. In contrast to OLF, CLF does not affect the superficial and deep layers of the ligamentum flavum and it occurs in degenerated and thickened ligaments with the calcified regions having no continuity with the lamina. These disease entities are best seen and diagnosed with computed tomography (CT) scans [6, 38, 39].

Rheumatoid Arthritis

Rheumatoid arthritis (RA) is an inflammatory disorder that commonly affects the cervical spine and is associated with females more than males (3:1 female-to-male ratio); however, men tend to have more severe cervical involvement in RA than women [40]. The prevalence of cervical spine abnormalities and cervical myelopathy in RA varies greatly and different ranges have been reported in the literature with cervical involvement ranging from 17% to 88% in RA patients and neurological complications ranging from 7% to 70% [40, 41].

The most common form of cervical involvement in RA is **atlantoaxial instability** and specifically anterior atlantoaxial subluxation (AAS) which occurs due to the laxity of primary and secondary ligamentous restraints, inflammation at the ligamentous insertion sites of the atlas and erosion of the odontoid process resulting in decreased space available for cord (SAC). Further damage occurs when a rheumatoid pannus forms from granulation tissue within the synovium destroying other spinal structures and further decreasing the SAC. As the SAC decreases in subluxation, the potential for cord compression and subsequent cervical myelopathy increases [41].

Neck pain is the most common complaint presenting in 40–80% of patients with RA involvement in the cervical spine [41]. MRI is the best modality at monitoring and diagnosing the severity of the RA cervical spine. Patients are neurologically evaluated using the Ranawat grading system for the rheumatoid spine (Table 6.2).

Spinal Tumors

Intradural extramedullary (IDEM) tumors or metastatic tumors to the cervical cord may cause external compression of the spinal cord and lead to cervical myelopathy. Primary IDEM

Table 6.2 Ranawat Classification for cervical myelopathy in rheumatoid arthritis patients [2, 41, 42]

Ranawat Grade	Severity of rheumatoid cervical spine
Class I	Normal or pain present but no neurological deficits
Class II	Subjective weakness, hyperreflexia, altered sensation
Class III a	Paresis (objective weakness), long tract signs but ambulatory
Class III b	Quadriparesis and non-ambulatory

tumors include meningiomas, neurofibromas, neurilemmomas, and schwannomas and are best diagnosed with Gadolinium-enhanced MRI. Primary IDEM tumors clinically present as Brown-Sequard type myelopathy as they typically compress the cord eccentrically. Metastasis to the cervical spine is less common compared to metastasis to other regions of the spinal cord as is commonly seen from primary tumors of the breast, prostate and lung [2].

Destructive Spondyloarthropathy

Destructive Spondyloarthropathy (DSA) or **Dialysis-related Spondyloarthropathy (DRSA)** is another cause of cervical myelopathy observed in patients receiving long term hemodialysis (10 or more years) and more commonly affects the cervical spine [43]. MRI of DSA patients shows amyloid deposition affecting the ligaments as well as atlantoaxial subluxation and odontoid destruction similar to the pathology in rheumatoid arthritis [44]. Possible pathophysiologic processes contributing to DSA include secondary hyperparathyroidism, microcrystal deposition, β2-microglobulin-associated amyloidosis, and aluminum intoxication [45].

Cervical Spine Anomalies of Congenital Disorders

Cervical spine anomalies associated with certain diseases can potentially lead to the compression of the spinal cord. There are numerous diseases associated with cervical spine anomalies including: Klippel-Feil Syndrome, Down Syndrome causing atlantoaxial instability, Morquio syndrome, Kniest syndrome, Goldenhar syndrome, Fibrodysplasia Ossificans, and others. Discussed below are some congenital disorders associated with cervical myelopathy [6].

Down Syndrome (DS) or trisomy 21 has been associated with cervical spine instability and can occur at the atlantoaxial and/or at the occiput-C1 levels with atlantoaxial instability occurring in

10–20% of DS patients. Cervical spine instability in Down syndrome patients rarely leads to symptoms with 1–2% of patients presenting with cervical myelopathy [46].

Klippel-Feil Syndrome (KFS) is a bone disorder that presents with a clinical triad of short neck, low posterior hairline, and restricted neck mobility and is diagnosed by radiographic imaging showing congenital fusion of cervical vertebrae. KFS is commonly sporadic but has been reported with other inheritance patterns and is associated with mutations in MEOX1 and GDF6 genes. KFS has been associated with cervical joint degeneration due to its direct vertebral involvement [6].

Morquio Disease (Mucopolysaccharidoses—MPS IV) is an autosomal recessive disease that causes glycosaminoglycans accumulation posterior to the dens, odontoid hypoplasia and atlantoaxial instability leading to severe myelopathy.

Larsen Syndrome is a rare autosomal dominant or autosomal recessive disease of the filamin B gene. Mutations in filamin B affect connective tissue which often causes developmental abnormalities of the spine such as cervical kyphosis and instability which increases the risk of spinal cord compression and cervical myelopathy.

Goldenhar Syndrome is caused by abnormal development of the first and second branchial arches and can result in vertebral anomalies with cervical involvement due to odontoid hypoplasia or basilar impression [47].

Pathophysiology

Cervical myelopathy develops over time as degenerative changes of the spine result in encroachment on the spinal cord and nearby structures. In adults, the cervical canal diameter is about 17–18 mm and the spinal cord diameter is about 10 mm [48]. With degeneration, the diameter of the canal reduces over time causing definite myelopathy at less than 6 mm disc cord space. The C5-C7 discal levels have increased mobility and, as a result, are the most affected levels of cord compression in the anterior-posterior axis [1]. Due to laxity of cervical vertebrae, anterolisthesis or retrolisthesis can also develop further implicating the myelopathy [49]. Compression of the spinal cord can result in demyelination, gliosis, myelomalacia, atrophy, exiting nerve root compression, and ischemia if the anterior spinal artery is involved [48, 49]. Many of the white matter tracts are also compressed which include the lateral corticospinal tracts, spinocerebellar tracts, spinothalamic tracts, posterior columns, as well as the dorsal nerve root itself. Clinical symptoms develop as a sequelae from the tracts affected. Voluntary skeletal muscle control is impaired from the lateral corticospinal tracts, proprioception is affected from the spinocerebellar tracts, pain and temperature is impaired by the spinothalamic tracts, position and vibration sense is impaired from the posterior columns, and dermatomal sensation is affected from the dorsal nerve root.

Signs and Symptoms

Symptoms of cervical myelopathy vary depending on the cervical levels involved, the etiology of the myelopathy, the anatomic structures involved, and the pathophysiological processes of disease. Neck pain or stiffness may manifest in structural disease caused by degeneration of discs and zygapophyseal joint arthritis. Symptoms of cervical stenosis from foraminal narrowing involve radiating arm pain, paresthesias, dysesthesias, numbness, and weakness of the upper extremities [1]. Cervical central canal stenosis can present with symptoms of the upper and lower extremities, neurogenic bladder or bowel, and unsteady gait along with weakness, paresthesias, or numbness of the lower extremities [1].

Since spinal cord compression can affect many of the white matter tracts, cervical myelopathy can present with both upper and lower motor neuron symptoms. Upper motor neuron involvement affects the lower extremities more than the upper extremities and causes hypertonic muscles, hyperreflexia, spastic paralysis, pronator drift, Babinski's sign, and Hoffman's sign [48–50]. Lower motor neuron affects the upper extremities more than the lower extremities causing hypotonic muscles, hyporeflexia, fasciculations, fibrillations, and flaccid paralysis [50]. Spinocerebellar tract involvement causes symptoms of ataxia and gait dysfunction due to proprioception disturbances. Posterior column involvement causes dysfunctions in deep touch, sensation, and vibration.

Clinically, patients will have upper extremity involvement more than lower extremity. Symptoms include numbness or tingling in the arms, fingers, and hands as well as weakness. Patients can have symptoms unilaterally or bilaterally [4]. Patients or their family members will notice them having difficulty grasping onto things and dropping items more frequently. Patients will experience difficulty with writing, buttoning shirts, and even eating. Patients can also present with falling more frequently due to balance problems and difficulty walking because of a wide based gait [50]. Some patients may lose the ability to walk at all. Some patients may also develop severe myelopathy that may lead to tetraplegia (Davies). Patients may also develop autonomic symptoms like urinary or bowel incontinence, urinary retention, or erectile dysfunction [4].

History

Patient's history is helpful for understanding what the possible cause of cervical myelopathy might be as well the anatomical structures involved by the symptoms presented. Onset of pain, any radiation of pain, recent trauma, associated symptoms provide the background to understanding etiology as well as appropriate treatment options.

Physical Exam

Neurological examinations are vital to assessing cervical myelopathy. Cerebellar involvement affecting regulation of balance, muscle tone, and coordination of voluntary movements should be assessed. The JOA Scale is a questionnaire that can be used to assess overall patient debilitation with six sections evaluating upper extremity motor, lower extremity motor, upper extremity sensory, lower extremity sensory, truncal sensory, and bladder function [2, 51].

The lower the score is, the more severe the disability. The Japanese Orthopedic Association Scale (Table 6.3) assesses the severity of cervical myelopathy with mild severity for a score > 13, moderate for scores of 9–13 and severe for scores <9 [52].

Table 6.3 Modified Japanese Orthopedic Association (mJOA) assesses the severity of cervical myelopathy [69]

Modified Japanese Orthopedic association (mJOA) score	
I. motor dysfunction score of the upper extremity	**Score**
Inability to move hands	0
Inability to eat with a spoon but able to move hands	1
Inability to button shirt but able to eat with spoon	2
Able to button shirt with great difficulty	3
Able to button shirt with slight difficulty	4
No dysfunction - Normal hand coordination	5
II. Motor dysfunction score of the lower extremity	**Score**
Complete loss of motor and sensory function	0
Sensory preservation with complete loss of movement	1
Able to move legs but unable to walk	2
Able to walk on flat floor with a walking aid (i.e., crane or crutch)	3
Able to walk up and/or down stairs with handrail	4
Moderate to significant lack of stability but able to walk up and/or down stairs without handrail	5
Mild lack of stability but can walk unaided with smooth reciprocation	6
No dysfunction - Normal walking	7
III. Sensory dysfunction of the upper extremity	**Score**
Complete loss of hand sensation	0
Severe sensory loss or pain	1
Mild sensory loss	2
No sensory loss	3
IV. Sphincter dysfunction score	**Score**
Inability to urinate voluntarily	0
Marked difficulty with micturition	1
Mild to moderate difficulty with micturition	2
Normal micturition	3

Mild myelopathy	mJOA from 15 to 17
Moderate myelopathy	mJOA from 12 to 14
Severe myelopathy	mJOA from 0 to 11

The Nurick scale is used to assess gait dysfunction (Table 6.4). Patient's ambulation should be observed for signs of ataxia as well as a wide based and staggering gait. Patients may have difficulty maintaining balance and can be seen holding onto nearby objects for support especially when asked to tandem walk.

Upper and lower motor symptoms should be evaluated. Lower motor findings will be found at the level of the compressive lesion and upper motor findings will be observed below the lesion [2]. Adduction and extension of the ulnar two or three fingers may become very weak known as "myelopathy hand." [2] Rapid alternating movements can also be impaired such as flipping one hand back and forth or opening and closing the fist. It takes a healthy person about 10 s to rapidly close and open a fist and 20 times which cannot be done in that time frame in patients with cervical myelopathy [48, 53].

Upper extremities should be evaluated for lower motor neuron symptoms of hyporeflexia, fasciculations, flaccid paralysis, and hypotonicity. The upper extremities should be examined for weakness due to atrophy of muscles and lack of coordination. Patients will have difficulty conducting motor tasks involving buttoning shirts or picking up small items due to muscle atrophy of the intrinsic and extrinsic hand muscles. Patients may complain of numbness of the hands causing them to drop things more frequently and limiting them from conducting their daily activi-

Table 6.4 Nurick Scale to assess gait dysfunction [70]

Nurick Grade	Definition
0	Signs or symptoms of root involvement but without evidence of spinal cord disease
1	Signs of spinal cord disease without difficulty in walking
2	Slight difficulty in walking that does not prevent full-time employment
3	Difficulty in walking that prevents full-time employment or daily tasks but does not require assistance with walking
4	Able to walk only with someone else's help or with the aid of a frame
5	Chair bound or bedridden

ties. Patients may complain of weakness making it difficult to carry objects. Patient's strength should be tested and evaluated. Reflex examinations of the biceps, brachioradialis, patellar, and Achilles will be hyperreflexic. If the u*pper and mid cervical spinal cord is involved, patients may have* upper motor neuron symptoms like *positive Hoffman sign and Romberg test* [50]. *Another reflex known as the "Scapulohumeral Reflex" is also seen in 95% of patients with lesions to the C3 vertebral body level in which tapping at the spine of the scapula or at the acromion in a caudal direction causes the scapula to elevate or the humerus to abduct* [2].

Lower extremities should be evaluated for upper motor neuron symptoms of hyperreflexia, weakness, muscle atrophy, spasticity, increased muscle tone, clonus, and Babinski sign. Assessment of the dorsal column involvement can be assessed with altered position and vibration sense. Patient's strength should be tested and evaluated.

Patients may complain of neck pain which can be assessed by testing range of motion. Patients will usually present with restricted motion in flexion and extension. Lhermitte sign can also be tested for by flexing the patient's neck which will produce electric-like sensation radiating down the torso when positive. Spurling sign can be assessed by extending the head, rotating, and applying pressure on inciting radicular pain [1].

Hypesthesia, paresthesia, or anesthesia should also be evaluated by sensory exams using dull and sharp objects as well as objects of different temperatures.

Diagnosis

What is the diagnostic approach and evaluation for cervical myelopathy?

Normally, the anterior-posterior measurement of the C3 through C7 spinal canal is 16–18 mm. With flexion, this diameter decreases by 2–3 mm and with extension may decrease it up to 3.5 mm [54, 55]. Absolute stenosis of the spinal canal is defined as a canal space less than 10 mm and relative spinal stenosis is

10–13 mm. The Torg ratio is measured to predict significant spinal stenosis to rule out any inherent radiographic measurement errors. This is calculated by dividing the sagittal diameter of the spinal canal by the sagittal diameter of the respective vertebral body and a ratio 0.8 or less is significant.

Cervical spine radiographs (X-rays) in AP and Lateral views are useful for evaluating the anatomy of the cervical spine and the progression of degenerative disease. These views portray neuroforaminal narrowing, spinal stenosis, loss of intervertebral disc space, facet abnormalities, uncovertebral joint arthropathy, and the degree of spondylolisthesis. Lateral views are useful to evaluate the posterior longitudinal ligament. Flexion-extension views are useful for evaluating ligamentous instability and can show anterolisthesis on flexion and retrolisthesis on extension. *The Torg-Pavlov ratio of 0.8 or less is used by dividing the anteroposterior diameter of the vertebral body by the anteroposterior diameter of the spinal canal to diagnose congenital spinal stenosis* [56].

Magnetic resonance imaging (MRI) is useful for evaluating the extent of spinal cord and nerve root compression as well as any soft tissue or osseous disease [57]. T1 and T2 weighted images are helpful to see compression and signal changes which are indicative of myelopathy. T1-weighted images show superior spatial resolution and T2-weighted images are helpful for evaluating the central canal and thecal sac [2].

Sagittal and axial cuts are used to evaluate discs, thickened ligamenta flava, cord anomalies, and severity of cord compression. Increased cord signal on T2 weighted images is helpful to determine the presence of edema, demyelination, myelomalacia, or gliosis [48].

Diffusion tensor imaging can portray the severity of cord injury before it can be seen on T2 images by detecting early damage to the myelin sheath. This scan has shown high sensitivity for detection of early cervical spondylotic myelopathy and intramedullary lesions [58, 59].

Computed tomographic myelography is used before surgery to depict the severity and location of neural compression. Use of CT is superior to MRI when distinguishing bone from soft tissue *intrusion into the cervical foramina for stenotic pathologic changes* [60].

Nerve conduction tests which include somatosensory evoked potentials are used to confirm myelopathy and electromyography is used to differentiate between peripheral and central nerve root involvement. Motor evoked potentials help differentiate between spinal cord compression and neurodegenerative disorders. Both SEPs and MEPs can also be used as markers of sensory and motor function during surgical treatment and rehabilitation [61].

Differential Diagnosis

What is the differential diagnosis for compressive cervical myelopathy?

The symptomatology of cervical myelopathy may present similarly in extrinsic vs. intrinsic causes as mentioned earlier in the chapter. The clinical significance of this classification is due to the importance of differentiating compressive cervical myelopathy from conditions of the nerve tissue itself. The differentials of compressive myelopathy have different treatments and prognosis and are important to consider when a patient presents with symptoms of cervical myelopathy. The differential diagnoses for compressive cervical myelopathy are listed in Table 6.5 [2].

Treatment and Management

What is the management and treatment for cervical myelopathy?

There are different modalities of treatment depending on the progress of disease. Patient's course can be unpredictable at times and follow a slow stepwise decline.

In the absence of clinical evidence of cervical myelopathy, patients are managed with conservative treatment and followed closely for biannual neurologic examinations and annual MRI tests. Patients should be instructed to make daily habit changes such as drinking from a straw to avoid extending the neck because hyperextending the neck can further compress the spinal cord.

Table 6.5 Differential Diagnosis for compressive/extrinsic cervical myelopathy—Adapted from Interventional Spine, Chapter 50 [2]

Viral infections
HIV-associated Vacuolar Myelopathy (AIDS-associated Myelopathy)
HTLV-I (Human T-cell Lymphotrophic Virus Type I) Associated Myelopathy (HAM) also known as Tropical Spastic Paraparesis (TSP)
Poliomyelitis due to polio virus
Intramedullary neoplasms
Astrocytoma
Ependymoma
Hemangioblastoma
Intraspinal Metastasis
Vascular diseases
Spinal Infarctions
Hematomyelia
Amyotrophic lateral sclerosis
Multiple Sclerosis
Vitamin B12 Deficiency
Syringomyelia
Radiation Myelopathy

Patients should also avoid any overhead activities for this reason [48, 62]. High risk activities such as horseback riding, contact sports, ladder climbing, and breaststroke swimming should be avoided [1]. In general, any hyperextension or hyperflexion activities should be avoided.

Physical activity is encouraged such as walking, stationary bicycling, and stretching. Static neck exercises are encouraged as well as strengthening the upper and lower extremities with resistance techniques. Patients are encouraged to feel steady and can be prescribed any assistive devices such as a cane or walker for walking. Pain can be managed with over the counter anti-inflammatory medications if needed. All fall precautions should be taken to prevent further injuries.

If patients display clinical evidence of cervical myelopathy, patients should be referred to a spine surgical specialist for an evaluation [1]. The cross-sectional area of the cord as well as the cord signal help determine whether surgery is indicated. If patients complain of pain, but not myelopathic symptoms, patients are advised to decrease physical activity for 2–3 days. If patients experience severe cervical or radicular pain, a soft neck collar is encouraged to be used for a few days [63]. Applying heat or ice packs can be therapeutic for some patients who experience radicular symptoms. Conservative pain management with acetaminophen and NSAIDs taken at regular intervals is encouraged. Increasing the pain regimen would require more than one family of NSAIDs to be completely ineffective or contraindicated. If pain is severe, opioids and muscle relaxants can be prescribed. Patients with severe and functionally limiting radicular symptoms may benefit from a taper dose of oral steroids for 7–10 days. None-remitting radicular pain can also be treated with gabapentin, pregabalin, tricyclic antidepressants, duloxetine, and others. Relieving depression and anxiety can also help relieve symptoms by medication, cognitive-behavioral therapy, biofeedback, self-hypnosis, and relaxation techniques.

Treatment

When conservative management fails, interlaminar or transforaminal epidural steroid injections can provide pain relief up to several months. If patients still do not respond, diagnostic medial branch nerve blocks and radiofrequency nerve ablation can provide relief. Some patients without significant central spinal canal stenosis are also candidates for spinal cord stimulator trial and implantation.

Symptom control of cervical myelopathy provides temporary relief and when the severity progresses, surgery should be considered. Surgery is not curative but can stop the progression of symptoms by increasing the canal space and lessening the cord compression. Although surgery comes with risks and can have serious complications, it can be very beneficial depending on the cause of the cervical myelopathy.

The Japanese Orthopaedic Association (JOA) classification system which evaluates the severity of spondylotic myelopathy as well as the Nurick scale which evaluates ambulatory function can be useful for determining the need for surgery. A JOA score of less than 13 with clinical symptoms and evidence of spinal cord compression on imaging is recommended for surgery [64]. Surgical options include decompressive single-level or multilevel laminectomy, laminoplasty, discectomy, foraminotomy, and cervical fusion by use of bone graft. Criteria for immediate surgical intervention include progressive weakness, bladder or bowel incontinence, unsteady gait, and upper motor neuron findings.

Patients who suffer from moderate to severe progressive CSM with significant cord compression or cord signal changes benefit from decompressive surgery which can be done from an anterior or posterior approach [48]. Patients with myelopathy that affects up to three spinal levels and patients with cervical kyphotic deformity benefit from the anterior approach which targets pathologic changes anterior to the spinal cord [64]. These anterior structures include the soft disc, hard disc, vertebral body spurs, and ossified posterior longitudinal ligament which can be removed without operating on the spinal cord [48]. Bone grafting and instrumentation ensure stabilization and fusion after the anterior cervical decompression and fusion.

The posterior approach consists of a laminectomy and laminoplasty giving access to hypertrophied laminae and ligamenta flava which is considered posterior disease. Laminectomies are less demanding than anterior corpectomies but can destabilize the cervical spine by pulling back the paraspinal muscles and resulting in loss of lordosis. Laminoplasty preserves the cervical facets and the laminae by increasing the sagittal canal diameter by lifting the laminae away from the degenerative site [65]. Unilateral or bilateral hinges allow symmetric expansion of the spinal canal which allows for the spinal cord to move and be decompressed.

Prognosis

Classifying the severity of cervical myelopathy is important to assess the efficacy of interventions. A variety of scales have been established and used in studies. More commonly used are the Nurick grading system and the Japanese Orthopedic Association system discussed previously in this chapter [66].

Early surgical intervention in cervical myelopathy patients, especially moderate and severe cases, has been associated with better clinical and neurological outcomes. Despite the poorer outcomes associated with delayed diagnosis and treatment of cervical myelopathy, studies have shown the diagnosis of Cervical Spondylotic Myelopathy frequently missed by primary care physicians who encounter the majority of patients initially presenting with cervical myelopathy symptoms [17].

More studies are needed to determine the effect of non-operative management on the clinical outcomes of cervical myelopathy. A systematic review showed that conservative management yielded poorer outcomes in moderate or severe cervical myelopathy patients. It showed that if non-operative management could have any beneficial effects in cervical myelopathy patients, it would be in mild forms of the disease. However, more studies are required to validate the effect of conservative management in mild cervical myelopathy with emphasis on the type on conservative management (e.g.: physical therapy, medications, injections, orthoses, traction, or a combination of treatments) [67].

Cervical myelopathy patients with underlying OPLL have also been noted to be at higher risk of worsening myelopathy with trauma and patients should be counseled on such a possibility [67].

It has also been shown that patients with a greater preoperative Nurick grade and symptoms for more than 12 months may have significantly lower odds of experiencing gait improvement or gait recovery after surgery for cervical myelopathy [68].

Conclusion

Cervical myelopathy is a compression of the spinal cord in the setting of either extrinsic factors, most commonly cervical stenosis or a cervical disc bulge, or intrinsic factors, which include viral infections, motor neuron disease or multiple sclerosis. When diagnosing cervical myelopathy a thorough neurological exam must be performed to detect any upper or lower motor neuron signs and to assess for gait dysfunction or impaired coordination. The treatment of cervical myelopathy is focused on symptomatic relief and strategies to arrest the progression of symptoms. Included among treatment these strategies are lifestyle modifications (avoiding activities that require hyperextension), oral analgesics, spinal injections and, if neurological deficits are present, surgery.

References

1. Meleger AL, Egyhazi R. Essentials of physical medicine and rehabilitation: musculoskeletal disorders, pain, and rehabilitation, chapter 7. Elsevier; 2015.
2. Kawaguchi Y. Interventional spine: an algorithmic approach, chapter 50: specific disorders. Saunders; 2007.
3. Kane SF, Abadie KV, Willson A. Degenerative cervical myelopathy: recognition and management. Am Fam Physician. 2020;102(12):740–50.
4. Davies BM, Mowforth OD, Smith EK, Kotter MR. Degenerative cervical myelopathy. BMJ. 2018:360.
5. Choi SH, Kang CN. Degenerative cervical myelopathy: pathophysiology and current treatment strategies. Asian Spine J. 2020;14(5):710.
6. Nouri A, Tetreault L, Singh A, Karadimas SK, Fehlings MG. Degenerative cervical myelopathy: epidemiology, genetics, and pathogenesis. Spine. 2015;40(12):E675–93.
7. Badhiwala JH, Ahuja CS, Akbar MA, Witiw CD, Nassiri F, Furlan JC, Curt A, Wilson JR, Fehlings MG. Degenerative cervical myelopathy— update and future directions. Nat Rev Neurol. 2020;16(2):108–24.
8. Potter K, Saifuddin A. MRI of chronic spinal cord injury. Br J Radiol. 2003;76(905):347–52.
9. Al-Mefty O, Harkey LH, Middleton TH, Smith RR, Fox JL. Myelopathic cervical spondylotic lesions demonstrated by magnetic resonance imaging. J Neurosurg. 1988;68(2):217–22.
10. Chen CJ, Lyu RK, Lee ST, Wong YC, Wang LJ. Intramedullary high signal intensity on T2-weighted MR images in cervical spondylotic myelopathy: prediction of prognosis with type of intensity. Radiology. 2001;221(3):789–94.
11. Vedantam A, Jonathan A, Rajshekhar V. Association of magnetic resonance imaging signal changes and outcome prediction after surgery for cervical spondylotic myelopathy. J Neurosurg Spine. 2011;15(6):660–6.
12. Tetreault LA, Dettori JR, Wilson JR, Singh A, Nouri A, Fehlings MG, Brodt ED, Jacobs WB. Systematic review of magnetic resonance imaging characteristics that affect treatment decision making and predict clinical outcome in patients with cervical spondylotic myelopathy. Spine. 2013;38(22S):S89–110.

13. Bakhsheshian J, Mehta VA, Liu JC. Current diagnosis and management of cervical spondylotic myelopathy. Global Spine J. 2017;7(6):572–86.
14. Iyer A, Azad TD, Tharin S. Cervical spondylotic myelopathy. Clin Spine Surg. 2016;29(10):408–14.
15. New PW, Cripps RA, Bonne LB. Global maps of non-traumatic spinal cord injury epidemiology: towards a living data repository. Spinal Cord. 2014;52(2):97–109.
16. Toledano M, Bartleson JD. Cervical spondylotic myelopathy. Neurol Clin. 2013;31(1):287–305.
17. Behrbalk E, Salame K, Regev GJ, Keynan O, Boszczyk B, Lidar Z. Delayed diagnosis of cervical spondylotic myelopathy by primary care physicians. Neurosurg Focus. 2013;35(1):E1.
18. Boogaarts HD, Bartels RH. Prevalence of cervical spondylotic myelopathy. Eur Spine J. 2015;24(2):139–41.
19. Rahimizadeh A, Asgari N, Soufiani H, Rahimizadeh S. Ossification of the cervical ligamentum flavum and case report with myelopathy. Surgical. Neurol Int. 2018;9
20. Kovalova I, Kerkovsky M, Kadanka Z, Kadanka Z Jr, Nemec M, Jurova B, Dusek L, Jarkovsky J, Bednarik J. Prevalence and imaging characteristics of nonmyelopathic and myelopathic spondylotic cervical cord compression. Spine. 2016;41(24):1908–16.
21. Bednarik J, Kadanka Z, Dusek L, Kerkovsky M, Vohanka S, Novotny O, Urbanek I, Kratochvilova D. Presymptomatic spondylotic cervical myelopathy: an updated predictive model. Eur Spine J. 2008;17(3):421–31.
22. Voorhies RM. Cervical spondylosis: recognition, differential diagnosis, and management. Ochsner J. 2001;3(2):78–84.
23. Park SJ, Kim SB, Kim MK, Lee SH, Oh IH. Clinical features and surgical results of cervical myelopathy caused by soft disc herniation. Korean J Spine. 2013;10(3):138.
24. O'Laoire SA, Thomas DG. Spinal cord compression due to prolapse of cervical intervertebral disc (herniation of nucleus pulposus): treatment in 26 cases by discectomy without interbody bone graft. J Neurosurg. 1983;59(5):847–53.
25. Boody BS, Lendner M, Vaccaro AR. Ossification of the posterior longitudinal ligament in the cervical spine: a review. Int Orthop. 2019;43(4):797–805.
26. Ehara S, Shimamura T, Nakamura R, Yamazaki K. Paravertebral ligamentous ossification: DISH, OPLL and OLF. Eur J Radiol. 1998;27(3):196–205.
27. Nouri A, Martin AR, Tetreault L, Nater A, Kato S, Nakashima H, Nagoshi N, Reihani-Kermani H, Fehlings MG. MRI analysis of the combined prospectively collected AOSpine North America and International Data: the prevalence and spectrum of pathologies in a global cohort of patients with degenerative cervical myelopathy. Spine. 2017;42(14):1058–67.

28. Maeda S, Koga H, Matsunaga S, Numasawa T, Ikari K, Furushima K, Harata S, Takeda J, Sakou T, Komiya S, Inoue I. Gender-specific haplotype association of collagen α2 (XI) gene in ossification of the posterior longitudinal ligament of the spine. J Hum Genet. 2001;46(1):1–4.
29. Yan L, Gao R, Liu Y, He B, Lv S, Hao D. The pathogenesis of ossification of the posterior longitudinal ligament. Aging Dis. 2017;8(5):570.
30. Abiola R, Rubery P, Mesfin A. Ossification of the posterior longitudinal ligament: etiology, diagnosis, and outcomes of nonoperative and operative management. Global spine J. 2016;6(2):195–204.
31. Bakhsh W, Saleh A, Yokogawa N, Gruber J, Rubery PT, Mesfin A. Cervical ossification of the posterior longitudinal ligament: a computed tomography–based epidemiological study of 2917 patients. Global Spine J 2019;9(8):820–825.
32. Fujimori T, Le H, Hu SS, Chin C, Pekmezci M, Schairer W, Tay BK, Hamasaki T, Yoshikawa H, Iwasaki M. Ossification of the posterior longitudinal ligament of the cervical spine in 3161 patients: a CT-based study. Spine. 2015;40(7):E394–403.
33. Stapleton CJ, Pham MH, Attenello FJ, Hsieh PC. Ossification of the posterior longitudinal ligament: genetics and pathophysiology. Neurosurg Focus. 2011;30(3):E6.
34. Matsunaga S, Sakou T. OPLL: disease entity, incidence, literature search, and prognosis. InOPLL 2006 (pp. 11-17). Springer, Tokyo.
35. Yoshimura N, Nagata K, Muraki S, Oka H, Yoshida M, Enyo Y, Kagotani R, Hashizume H, Yamada H, Ishimoto Y, Teraguchi M. Prevalence and progression of radiographic ossification of the posterior longitudinal ligament and associated factors in the Japanese population: a 3-year follow-up of the ROAD study. Osteoporos Int. 2014;25(3):1089–98.
36. Hollenberg AM, Mesfin A. Ossification of the posterior longitudinal ligament in north American patients: does presentation with spinal cord injury matter? World Neurosurg. 2020;143:e581–9.
37. Tsuyama NA. Ossification of the posterior longitudinal ligament of the spine. Clin Orthop Relat Res. 1984;1(184):71–84.
38. Miyasaka K, Kaneda K, Sato S, Iwasaki Y, Abe S, Takei H, Tsuru M, Tashiro K, Abe H, Fujioka Y. Myelopathy due to ossification or calcification of the ligamentum flavum: radiologic and histologic evaluations. Am J Neuroradiol. 1983;4(3):629–32.
39. Meyer CA, Vagal AS, Seaman D. Put your back into it: pathologic conditions of the spine at chest CT. Radiographics. 2011;31(5):1425–41.
40. Nguyen HV, Ludwig SC, Silber J, Gelb DE, Anderson PA, Frank L, Vaccaro AR. Rheumatoid arthritis of the cervical spine. Spine J. 2004;4(3):329–34.
41. Wasserman BR, Moskovicich R, Razi AE. Rheumatoid arthritis of the cervical spine. Bull NYU Hosp Joint Dis. 2011;69:136–48.

42. Ranawat CS, O'Leary PA, Pellicci PA, Tsairis PE, Marchisello PE, Dorr LA. Cervical spine fusion in rheumatoid arthritis. J Bone Joint Surg Am. 1979;61(7):1003–10.
43. Kuntz D, Naveau B, Bardin T, Drueke T, Treves R, Dryll A. Destructive spondylarthropathy in hemodialyzed patients. Arthritis Rheum. 1984;27(4):369–75.
44. Shiota E, Naito M, Tsuchiya K. Surgical therapy for dialysis-related spondyloarthropathy: review of 30 cases. Clin Spine Surg. 2001;14(2):165–71.
45. Bindi P, Chanard J. Destructive spondyloarthropathy in dialysis patients: an overview. Nephron. 1990;55(2):104–9.
46. Ali FE, Al-Bustan MA, Al-Busairi WA, Al-Mulla FA, Esbaita EY. Cervical spine abnormalities associated with Down syndrome. Int Orthop. 2006;30(4):284–9.
47. McKay SD, Al-Omari A, Tomlinson LA, Dormans JP. Review of cervical spine anomalies in genetic syndromes. Spine. 2012;37(5):E269–77.
48. Fast A, Dudkiewicz I. Essentials of physical medicine and rehabilitation: musculoskeletal disorders, pain, and rehabilitation, chapter 1, cervical Spondylotic myelopathy. Elsevier; 2015.
49. Rao R. Neck pain, cervical radiculopathy, and cervical myelopathy: pathophysiology, natural history, and clinical evaluation. JBJS. 2002;84(10):1872–81.
50. McCartney S, Baskerville R, Blagg S, McCartney D. Cervical radiculopathy and cervical myelopathy: diagnosis and management in primary care. Br J Gen Pract. 2018;68(666):44–6.
51. Donnally CJ III, Butler AJ, Rush AJ III, Bondar KJ, Wang MY, Eismont FJ. The most influential publications in cervical myelopathy. J Spine Surg. 2018;4(4):770.
52. Yonenobu K, Abumi K, Nagata K, Taketomi E, Ueyama K. Interobserver and intraobserver reliability of the Japanese Orthopaedic Association scoring system for evaluation of cervical compression myelopathy. Spine. 2001;26(17):1890–4.
53. Ono K, Ebara S, Fuji TA, Yonenobu KA, Fujiwara KE, Yamashita KA. Myelopathy hand. New clinical signs of cervical cord damage. J Bone Joint Surg. 1987;69(2):215–9.
54. Penning L. Functional radiographic examination. Functional pathology of the cervical spine. Penning, pp. 1–27.
55. Gu R, Zhu Q, Lin Y, Yang X, Gao Z, Tanaka Y. Dynamic canal encroachment of ligamentum flavum: an in vitro study of cadaveric specimens. Clin Spine Surg. 2006;19(3):187–90.
56. Cantu RC. The cervical spinal stenosis controversy. Clin Sports Med. 1998;17(1):121–6.
57. Nouri A, Martin AR, Mikulis D, Fehlings MG. Magnetic resonance imaging assessment of degenerative cervical myelopathy: a review of struc-

tural changes and measurement techniques. Neurosurg Focus. 2016;40(6):E5.
58. Rajasekaran S, Kanna RM, Shetty AP. Diffusion tensor imaging of the spinal cord and its clinical applications. J Bone Joint Surg Br. 2012;94(8):1024–31.
59. Song T, Chen WJ, Yang B, Zhao HP, Huang JW, Cai MJ, Dong TF, Li TS. Diffusion tensor imaging in the cervical spinal cord. Eur Spine J. 2011;20(3):422–8.
60. Del Grande F, Maus TP, Carrino JA. Imaging the intervertebral disk: age-related changes, herniations, and radicular pain. Radiol Clin. 2012;50(4):629–49.
61. Nardone R, Höller Y, Brigo F, Frey VN, Lochner P, Leis S, Golaszewski S, Trinka E. The contribution of neurophysiology in the diagnosis and management of cervical spondylotic myelopathy: a review. Spinal Cord. 2016;54(10):756–66.
62. Lauryssen C, Riew KD, Wang JC. Severe cervical stenosis: operative treatment of continued conservative care. Spine Line. 2006;8(1):21–5.
63. Persson LC, Carlsson CA, Carlsson JY. Long-lasting cervical radicular pain managed with surgery, physiotherapy, or a cervical collar: a prospective, randomized study. Spine. 1997;22(7):751–8.
64. Bono CM, Fisher CG, editors. Prove it! Evidence-based analysis of common spine practice. Lippincott Williams & Wilkins; 2010.
65. Hirabayashi K, Watanabe K, Wakano K, Suzuki N, Satomi K, Ishii Y. Expansive open-door laminoplasty for cervical spinal stenotic myelopathy. Spine. 1983;8(7):693–9.
66. Kim DH, Vaccaro AR. Interventional spine: an algorithmic approach, chapter 70: surgical treatment of cervical myelopathy. Saunders; 2007.
67. Rhee JM, Shamji MF, Erwin WM, Bransford RJ, Yoon ST, Smith JS, Kim HJ, Ely CG, Dettori JR, Patel AA, Kalsi-Ryan S. Nonoperative management of cervical myelopathy: a systematic review. Spine. 2013;38(22S):S55–67.
68. De la Garza-Ramos R, Ramhmdani S, Kosztowski T, Xu R, Yassari R, Witham TF, Bydon A. Prognostic value of preoperative nurick grade and time with symptoms in patients with cervical myelopathy and gait impairment. World Neurosurg. 2017;105:314–20.
69. Benzel EC, Lancon J, Kesterson L, Hadden T. Cervical laminectomy and dentate ligament section for cervical spondy- lotic myelopathy. J Spinal Disord. 1991;4(3):286–95.
70. Nurick S. The pathogenesis of the spinal cord disorder associated with cervical spondylosis. Brain. 1972;95:87–100.

Sports Trauma and Fractures

Rebecca Freedman and Irene Kalbian

Introduction

Cervical spine injuries in athletics can be seen in both collision and non-collision sports. However, injury patterns can range from relatively minor and temporary injuries, to nerve injuries, to stable fractures with no neurological involvement, and to unstable, life-threatening spinal cord injuries. Catastrophic spinal injuries in sport are most likely to occur in the cervical spine due to straight axial compression to the vertex of the head and compression-flexion forces. These mechanisms of injury are seen in sports such as American football, ice hockey, rugby, wrestling, gymnastics, and diving. Catastrophic injuries can result in severe injury with no permanent disability, permanent severe functional disability, or even fatality [1]. Fortunately, catastrophic cervical spine injuries rarely occur, and improved education, sporting rules, and player techniques have significantly decreased the rates of severe injuries. Regardless, every suspected cervical injury sustained during sport should be expeditiously and thoroughly evaluated and managed. It is imperative for both on-field and off-field medical per-

R. Freedman (✉) · I. Kalbian
Department of Rehabilitation and Human Performance, Icahn School of Medicine at Mount Sinai, New York, NY, USA

© The Author(s), under exclusive license to Springer Nature Switzerland AG 2022
M. Harbus et al. (eds.), *A Case-Based Approach to Neck Pain*,
https://doi.org/10.1007/978-3-031-17308-0_7

sonnel to be knowledgeable about the spectrum and mechanisms of cervical spine injuries. In this chapter, we review acute cervical spine traumas and injuries.

Epidemiology

Sports trauma accounts for roughly 8% of the 17,900 new spinal cord injuries (SCI) per year in the USA [2]. Sports-related SCIs most frequently occur in the cervical spine with about 84% of all sports-related SCIs resulting in tetraplegia [2, 3]. Epidemiological data shows that cervical injury is, by far, the leading cause of SCI worldwide for ice hockey, skiing, diving, and American football, and constitutes a large percentage of SCI in rugby [4]. Most commonly, SCIs are seen in athletes 30 years old or younger [5], with diving as the major contributing sport to SCIs [2].

Many sports place athletes at a proportionally higher risk for sustaining a catastrophic cervical spine injury such as American football, hockey, wrestling, rugby, skiing, gymnastics, baseball, and cheerleading [1, 6]. Among high school and college sports participants, 48.6% of traumatic (direct) catastrophic injuries occur to the spine, with spine fractures occurring most commonly, followed by SCI without spine fracture, then SCI with a fracture [1]. The vast majority of cervical spine injuries occur via contact mechanisms. Direct traumatic injury can be due to contact with another player, the apparatus, or the ground/surface. For instance, it has been reported that wrestlers are more likely to sustain a cervical spine injury due to contact with the playing surface, whereas the most common mechanism of injury in American football players is due to contact with another player [6]. Hockey players, on the other hand, are more likely to sustain a cervical spine injury due to checking from behind into the boards. The rate of neck injuries is found to be higher during competition than in practice [1, 6, 7]. It is also important to note that the mechanisms involved in catastrophic cervical spine injuries can result in injuries to the cervical nerve roots, cervical discs, and brachial plexus.

Overall, muscle injuries to the cervical spine are reported most frequently, and nerve injuries are the most common cause of severe cervical spine injury [6].

Notoriously, American football records the largest number of direct traumatic catastrophic injuries, particularly in high school and college sports largely due to the nature of the sport and the number of participants [1, 6]. The most frequent activity which leads to a direct traumatic injury is tackling or being tackled [2]. However, the incidence of catastrophic cervical injuries has markedly declined since the 1970s due to notable rule changes, such as the banning of spearing in 1976 (tackling another player with the crown of the head) [8, 9]. Similarly, rugby and ice hockey have implemented new rules to prohibit dangerous plays that increase the risk of sustaining a traumatic, direct cervical injury [4, 10, 11]. A large proportion of American football injuries to the cervical spine remain nerve-related whereas in boys' ice hockey, cervical fractures represent a greater proportion of neck injuries [6].

Although safety measures continue to be implemented, cervical spine injury is still a risk across all sports.

Cervical Spine Fractures and Dislocations

Unstable Fractures and Dislocation

Definition and Mechanism of Injury

A cervical spine fracture is deemed unstable when the structural integrity of the vertebral column is disrupted, impairing normal physiologic motion and resulting in injury with actual or potential damage to the spinal cord [12]. The most common mechanism resulting in unstable cervical spine injuries is axial loading, at which time the neck is often in a straightened or flexed position, compromising the usual slightly lordotic alignment of the cervical spine. Biomechanically, this alters the normal dissipation of forces from the paravertebral muscles and intervertebral discs into the cervical column. Under these forces the spine can fail, placing the spine and cord at risk for injury. Axial compression is the most frequent cause of unstable cervical fracture in ice hockey and American football leading to spinal cord injury [9, 11].

Unstable fractures or dislocations of the lower cervical spine are the most common traumatic cause of catastrophic cervical spine injuries in collision sport athletes. As the spinal canal is narrowest from C4 to C7, an injury to this region is more likely to result in a SCI. In comparison, fractures of the upper cervical spine are uncommon. Relative frequency varies by sport, however, upper cervical injuries are consistently more rare than lower cervical injuries [13, 14]. Traumatic conditions most likely to result in upper cervical cord injury are those that destabilize the atlantoaxial complex.

Lower Cervical Spine Fractures

Flexion Teardrop Fracture

A flexion teardrop fracture can result from compression-flexion forces to the subaxial cervical spine. The compression is transmitted along the longitudinal axis of the straightened or flexed spine. The resulting tensile forces disrupt the posterior spinal ligaments, leading to anterior column shortening and posterior column lengthening, and retropulsion of the fractured vertebral body into the spinal canal [15]. For example, teardrop fractures are seen when axial forces are applied by an oncoming player to the vertex of an opponent's helmet, while the neck is prepositioned in flexion [15]. This pattern of injury is also prevalent in non-collision sports such as diving. In a small study of 65 divers with vertebral lesions, 61% experienced a teardrop fracture [16]. The flexion teardrop fracture results in significant structural instability and is frequently associated with injury to the spinal cord, including but not limited to anterior cord syndrome.

Burst Fracture

A burst fracture is another prevalent fracture type seen in collision sports, resulting from a high-impact, pure compressive force at the top of an athlete's head. For example, in helmeted athletes, axial forces are applied by an oncoming body to the vertex of a player's helmet, while the neck is in a neutral alignment with slight extension of the cervical spine. The anterior and posterior columns both shorten and intra-disc pressure increases until the vertebra fails, resulting in comminution of the vertebral body. Bone fragments are subsequently displaced in all directions into surrounding structures, and spinal cord injury most often results from the retropulsion of bone into the spinal canal [15]. Burst fractures are seen in multiple collision sports including wrestling, rugby, American football, and ice hockey [9, 11, 17, 18]. They have also been reported with diving accidents, with Aito et al. finding that 21% of divers with vertebral lesions experienced a burst fracture [16].

Facet Joint Dislocations

Facet joint dislocations are another source of catastrophic cervical spine injury and occur due to flexion forces. The traumatic event usually comprises a direct blow to the head or a rapid deceleration of the torso leading to disruption of the stabilizing spinal ligaments. Bilateral facet dislocation is frequently associated with spinal cord injury. A study of cervical spine injuries in rugby players identified facet joint dislocations, particularly bilateral facet dislocations at C4-C5 and C5-C6 motion segments, as the most common cervical spine injury in rugby players [19]. Unilateral facet dislocation can result when axial rotation is added to the flexion impact force, though unilateral dislocations are generally stable and do not place the spinal cord at risk [15].

Presentation

Athletes who experience a catastrophic lower cervical spine injury resulting in SCI exhibit a wide range of neurologic symptoms. Neurological dysfunction may range from quadriplegia below the lesion to incomplete spinal cord injury syndromes like central cord syndrome or anterior cord syndrome [15]. Central cord syndrome results in weakness greater in the upper extremities than the lower extremities as well as decreased sensation. Anterior cord syndrome is characterized by loss of pain and temperature at and below the level of the lesion, as well as variable loss of motor function below the level of the lesion.

Evaluation and Management

Initial evaluation of any suspected unstable cervical spine injury includes neurological assessment (in addition to proper on-field management, stabilization, and immobilization). This is followed by imaging studies (X-ray, CT, and MRI) to ascertain for bony and ligamentous injury as well as any associated cord damage. A comprehensive understanding of patient and injury specific factors such as additional medical conditions, neurological compromise, injury mechanism, and degree of instability is key to formulating the appropriate treatment plan [20]. That being said, management of unstable lower cervical spine fractures is generally surgical.

Return to Play

Athletes, who underwent a one-level anterior cervical discectomy and fusion, have a history of a healed, nondisplaced cervical fracture with no malalignment, or underwent a one-level cervical fusion have no contraindications to return to play [15]. Torg et al. outlined relative and absolute contraindications to return to play after cervical fracture that have been widely adopted [9]. Prior upper cervical spine fracture(s) is a relative contraindication requiring further evaluation on the individual athlete level, including neurological status, resultant degree of instability, and comorbid medical conditions [20]. Furthermore, a healed two-level fusion is a relative contraindication. Absolute contraindications to return to play include the following: history of C1-C2 cervical fusion, acute posterior element or cervical body fracture regardless of ligamentous involvement, healed subaxial spine fracture with residual kyphosis, three-level cervical fusion, status-post cervical laminectomy, or radiological evidence of distraction-extension on radiographic study [9]. Cervical spinal cord abnormality on MRI is an absolute contraindication to returning participation in contact sports [16].

Upper Cervical Spine Fractures

Odontoid Fracture

Odontoid fractures are the most common fractures of the C2 dens. There are three types of odontoid fractures: Type I is a fracture of the upper part of the odontoid (potentially unstable); Type II is a fracture of the base of the odontoid (unstable); and Type III is a fracture through the odontoid and the lateral masses of the C2 vertebra (best prognosis for healing). Fracture of the odontoid and rupture of the transverse atlantal ligament destabilize the atlantoaxial complex. Dodwell et al. found that in athletes, odontoid fractures are the most common upper cervical spine injury. Odontoid fractures tend to occur in a biphasic age distribution in young adults and the elderly. They are observed in young adults (ages 20–30) in high-energy impact traumas such as American football and diving accidents [21]. Standard lateral and open-mouth odontoid radiographs can assist in diagnosis.

Jefferson Fracture

A Jefferson fracture is a burst fracture specifically of the atlas, resulting from a vertical compression force. The fracture occurs through both the C1 anterior and posterior arches and disrupts the transverse atlantal ligament. While not commonly reported in the literature, there are case reports of Jefferson fractures occurring in American football players during head-to-chest collisions [22, 23]. Jefferson fractures are not always unstable as the fracture increases the dimensions of the spinal canal, but if a shard of bone reaches the spinal cord it can cause cord injury [15].

Hangman's Fracture

A hangman's fracture is characterized by traumatic bilateral fracture of the pars interarticularis of the axis. The mechanism of injury is an extension force causing traumatic spondylolisthesis of the axis. As with Jefferson fractures, hangman's fractures are not always unstable, but often the traumatic spondylolisthesis causes a shard of bone to injure the spinal cord [15]. Loebel et al.

reported on a case of a hangman's fracture in a semi-professional parachuter, occurring when the parachute opened improperly and resulted in an abrupt deceleration in the air. Although uncommon, hangman's fracture has also been seen in diving accidents where the entry is complicated by extension forces on the head and neck [24].

Presentation

Spinal cord damage and neurologic dysfunction is uncommon in upper cervical spine injury because proportionately greater space is available within the upper spinal canal compared to lower segments. When symptoms do occur they can be severe including quadriplegia and diaphragmatic paralysis with acute respiratory insufficiency resulting from trauma to the phrenic nerve roots [15].

Evaluation and Management

Initial evaluation of suspected unstable upper cervical spine injury is identical to that in lower cervical spine injury. This includes neurological assessment, imaging studies, and integration of patient specific factors [20]. As with lower cervical spine fractures, accurate and timely diagnosis and stabilization of the craniocervical junction remains the guiding principle for optimal outcomes.

Treatment is a subject of debate and varies by fracture type. Highly unstable injuries like atlanto-occipital dissociations or injuries resulting in C1-C2 instability necessitate surgical stabilization. In most cases an odontoid fracture can be treated with a hard cervical collar or a halo vest. Exceptions to this include odontoid fractures associated with neurologic dysfunction or significant displacement, which would require surgical intervention such as arthrodesis or screw fixation [25]. Jefferson fracture treatment varies based on fracture pattern but can require surgical stabilization. Hangman's fractures of the axis are generally treated conservatively, but reduction and fusion are utilized for atypical patterns and displaced fractures that risk cord injury [26].

Return to Play

Return to play following upper cervical fractures is guided by the same criteria for lower cervical fractures by Torg et al. [9], as outlined in the section above.

Stable Fractures and Dislocations

Definition and Mechanism of Injury

Spinous Process Fracture

Cervical spinous process fractures are often an isolated finding, most commonly seen in the lower cervical spine or upper thoracic spine. One mechanism of injury is a direct hit to the spinous process which can occur in collision sports. A second mechanism is avulsion of the spinous process by intraspinous and supraspinous ligaments during forced cervical spine hyperextension or hyperflexion. This is seen with high velocity trauma particularly in American football. A spinous process fracture at C7 is known as a clay shoveler's fracture which occurs following a flexion force [15].

Wedge Fracture

Wedge fractures occur when a compression force crushes the anterior portion of the vertebral body, forming a wedge. This is seen in diving accidents with improper water entry, as well as horseback riding when riders are thrown from their horse [17, 27].

Presentation

Stable fractures refer to cervical injuries that do not result in structural disruption of the vertebral column and thus the spinal cord remains protected. Fractures of the spinous process most often present with posterior neck pain as well as possible bruising and swelling, but are not associated with neurological deficits. With wedge fractures the surrounding ligaments generally remain intact and neurological damage is rare, but there is significant soft tissue swelling associated with the injury [15].

Evaluation and Management

Stable fractures can be treated conservatively by limiting range of motion and thereby minimizing pain. This is best accomplished with a soft cervical orthosis for 4–6 weeks while the fracture heals. Repeat radiographs in flexion and extension should be performed prior to allowing range of motion to reassess stability [15].

Return to Play

Return to play is guided by symptom resolution and repeat radiographs demonstrating a healed fracture [15].

Congenital Spinal Anomalies

Certain congenital spinal anomalies can place athletes at great risk for spinal cord injury if participating in collision sports. These abnormalities alter the structural integrity of the spinal column and its ability to distribute forces upon loading. Klippel-Feil syndrome is a lower cervical spine anomaly, in which there is a fusion of two or more vertebrae due to failure of segmentation. This reduces the overall motion of the spine, impeding the spine from properly dissipating forces. Furthermore, there is increased stress on the adjacent segments which can result in degenerative stenosis or mechanical instability [28]. Another group of athletes with increased risk of severe spinal cord injury during athletics are those who have Down syndrome. Atlantoaxial and/or atlanto-occipital instability has been found in up to 15% of these patients [24, 29]. Any instability prohibits these athletes from participating in high-risk activities that could cause hyperflexion or hyperextension to the cervical spine. Screening is mandated by the Special Olympics Inc. [29] Other conditions with atlantoaxial and atlanto-occipital instability include Ehlers-Danlos syndrome, Marfan syndrome, os odontoideum, and juvenile rheumatoid arthritis.

Non-fracture or Dislocation Cervical Spine-Related Trauma

Cervical Cord Neurapraxia

Definition and Mechanism of Injury
Cervical cord neurapraxia (CCN) is a temporary episode of neurological symptoms, which may involve sensory and/or motor deficits to both arms, both legs, all four extremities, or an ipsilateral arm and leg [9]. It is most commonly seen in contact sports such as American football, ice hockey, and wrestling, however, it can happen in any sport where collisions occur, with other athletes or with equipment. Typically, this injury results from cervical spine hyperextension or hyperflexion (both of which narrow the spinal canal) or axial loading. When the spinal cord becomes temporarily stretched or compressed, there is a transient alteration in nervous function below the level of injury, producing paresthesias, and/or weakness [9].

Congenital or degenerative cervical canal stenosis can predispose athletes for CCN and recurrent episodes. Excessive flexion or extension causes further narrowing of the spinal canal, compressing the cord against boney or ligamentous structures [9]. Athletes with spear tackler's spine, defined as the development of stenosis of the cervical canal with the loss of the normal cervical lordosis from repeated axial compression, are also at increased risk for transient (and permanent) spinal cord injury [30].

Presentation
Athletes will experience acute, transient sensory changes with or without motor changes in both arms, both legs, all four extremities, or an ipsilateral arm and leg. Sensory symptoms can include burning, numbness, or tingling. Motor symptoms can include weakness or paralysis. Typically the cervical spine bony structure is uninjured and the athlete is pain-free at time of injury [13]. Symptoms will last anywhere from less than 15 minutes to as long as 48 hours [9]. Usually, an athlete will regain full function and cervical range of motion as symptoms subside.

Evaluation and Management

Plain radiographs of the cervical spine in flexion and extension should be obtained if the patient is neurologically stable. Further imaging including magnetic resonance imaging (MRI) should be performed to assess for intrinsic spinal cord abnormalities, stenosis or ongoing spinal cord or nerve root compression. MRI may also reveal a disc herniation or disc-osteophyte complex causing a narrowed spinal canal and functional spinal stenosis. Any athlete with neurological symptoms present in more than one limb, even if transient, should undergo a cervical spine MRI to evaluate for a potential source of the symptoms [30].

The Torg or Torg-Pavlov ratio is derived from lateral cervical spine radiographs comparing the sagittal diameter of the spinal canal to the midbody diameter of the vertebral body at the same level. A ratio of less than 0.8 has been found to be predictive of spinal stenosis [9]. Although it has a high sensitivity rate, it has a low positive predictive value, and is not recommended for use as a routine screening tool in asymptomatic athletes. In comparison, measuring functional spinal stenosis can be more useful. Functional spinal stenosis is seen when there is a loss of the normal amount of cerebrospinal fluid (CSF) around the spinal cord on MRI or CT myelography. The functional reserve refers to how much CSF is able to flow freely around the spinal cord. Decreased CSF around the spinal cord, or in more severe cases a cord defect, is indicative of more significant stenosis [30].

Return to Play

Guidelines for return to play after cervical cord neurapraxia in asymptomatic athletes vary in recommendations, as long-term data is not widely available. An episode of uncomplicated CCN (with normal radiographs, normal MRI with no evidence of functional spinal stenosis, and no cervical laxity) is not an absolute contraindication for returning to contact sports. Symptoms should, however, completely resolve prior to returning to play [9, 30, 31]. It is important to educate athletes on the risk factors that predispose to CCN and the risks of returning to contact sports.

If athletes with an uncomplicated CCN are found to have degenerative joint disease, intervertebral disc disease or other radiologic findings which can cause a narrowed spinal canal or spinal stenosis, returning to contact sports is a relative contraindication.

Generally, absolute contraindications include cervical fracture or ligamentous injury, recurrent episodes, any persistent neurological signs or symptoms, and MRI evidence of cord signal changes or edema [9, 13]. However, it has also been suggested that functional spinal stenosis seen on MRI after an episode of CCN be an absolute contraindication for returning to contact sport because athletes have an increased risk of CCN and permanent neurologic injury [32].

Patients without spinal instability can return to contact sport activities without increased risk of permanent neurological injury, however, the overall recurrence rate is strongly correlated to functional spinal stenosis and the degree of narrowing of the cervical canal [9].

Stinger/Burners

Definition and Mechanism of Injury

Stingers, also known as burners, are transient unilateral radiculopathies or brachial plexopathies, resulting from trauma to the cervical nerve roots or brachial plexus. They are the most common cervical neurologic injury in athletes. There are three proposed mechanisms of injury for athletes who sustain a stinger: (1) a traction injury, which occurs when the neck is forced into lateral flexion while the contralateral shoulder is depressed, such as in a tackle, stretching the cervical nerve roots and the brachial plexus; (2) compressive injuries which occur when the neck is forced into extension and lateral flexion, compressing the cervical nerve roots by narrowing the neural foramen; and (3) direct compression to the brachial plexus at Erb's point, located superior to the clavicle [30, 33, 34].

Transient brachial plexopathies and radiculopathies classically occur in collision athletes due to the nature of the sport, such as rugby and American football, but they can also occur in gymnastics, wrestling, weight lifting, and boxing. Stingers were reported to be the most common cervical injury among NCAA American football players [35]. A study found that 50.4% of existing collegiate American football players had experienced multiple stingers throughout their careers [36]. Similarly, more than one-third of all rugby players experience a burner or stinger in a single season [37].

Several studies have also demonstrated a higher incidence of stingers and recurrences in athletes with cervical spondylosis, degenerative disc disease, and narrowing of the intervertebral foramina, as this predisposes the nerve roots to injury [38–40]. Chronic stingers, in comparison to acute stingers, are more likely when long-term structural changes in the subaxial cervical spinal canal exist.

Presentation

Athletes with stingers will experience a transient episode of unilateral upper extremity pain and/or paresthesias, with possible associated weakness. Immediately after a high-impact collision, an athlete may shake their arm or have it hanging by their side, with complaints of burning or numbness in the affected extremity. Athletes may also hold their head in a slight lateral flexion to relieve pressure on the irritated nerve root in its foramen [15]. The duration of symptoms can vary, lasting anywhere from seconds to minutes, or even days to weeks. Motor symptoms can often have a delayed presentation relative to sensory.

Most commonly, symptoms will present in the C5 and C6 sensory and motor distribution due to the increased susceptibility for injury to the upper trunk of the brachial plexus. However, pain may be non-dermatomal in presentation. Weakness may be detected in the deltoid, supraspinatous, infraspinatous, biceps, brachioradialis, pronator teres, or wrist extensors. Athletes may have impaired strength in shoulder abduction, shoulder external rotation, elbow flexion and wrist extension. Athletes may also have a positive Spurling's maneuver [34].

Importantly, stingers are exclusively unilateral. Therefore, athletes who present with burning, numbness or tingling in both of their arms or hands, or report symptoms in their lower extremities, should be promptly evaluated for a spinal cord injury.

Evaluation and Management

If an athlete has any persistent neurological symptoms or painful cervical neck range of motion, imaging is warranted to evaluate for underlying anatomical pathologies predisposing the athlete to injury. As previously mentioned, chronic or recurrent stingers are often associated with spondylosis, neural foraminal narrowing or cervical disc disease. Cervical radiographs can identify any bony foraminal narrowing or instability in flexion and extension. MRI can further evaluate for disc herniations or disc-osteophyte complexes that may be contributing to any neural foraminal narrowing or nerve root compression, especially in athletes with symptoms lasting longer than 1 hour, weakness, or symptoms in a particular nerve root distribution [30]. A brachial plexus MRI can also be completed if persistent symptoms are suspected to stem from the brachial plexus. Electrodiagnostic testing (EDX) can also be considered in athletes with persistent symptoms. EDX can help localize a cervical nerve root injury or a brachial plexus injury, and EDX findings can help define the severity of injury (i.e., neurapraxia versus more severe neurological injury) and predicted prognosis timeline.

Stinger management is largely based upon the mechanism of injury and severity of symptoms, but most are treatable through supportive care and rehabilitation. Therapy programs should focus on cervical musculature strength and flexibility imbalances, postural correction, and general strengthening [41]. Although cervical collars are occasionally used with the goal of limiting extension and lateral bending, data regarding their utility in preventing stingers is lacking [30, 31].

Return to Play

Stingers are normally self-limited. Although there are no standardized protocols for returning to play, complete resolution of symptoms with full, pain-free cervical range of motion, a normal neurological exam, and full upper extremity strength are required prior to returning to contact athletic activity. Athletes who sustain an isolated episode of a stinger with rapid resolution of symptoms and a normal neurological examination can return to play in the same game without further diagnostic work up [42]. This applies to a first time episode or a repeated episode in separate seasons. If an athlete experiences three or more recurrent stingers with rapid resolution of symptoms and a normal neurological examination in separate seasons, a thorough evaluation, including imaging, is recommended before returning to contact sports.

If repeated episodes occur in the same game, an athlete should be removed from competition and undergo thorough evaluation even if symptoms resolve. It is recommended that athletes do not return to play if three or more stingers occur within 1 year without further medical intervention and imaging [43]. As previously mentioned, athletes with repeated stingers have a higher prevalence of cervical spondylosis, which predisposes them for further cervical spine injuries. Any stinger with persistent neurological deficits always necessitates a thorough evaluation including imaging prior to returning to contact sports. Absolute contraindications include evidence of a cervical disc herniation, cervical bony anomalies, or cervical instability on imaging, persistent weakness, evidence of myelopathy, continued pain, or reduced cervical range of motion. Cervical spinal stenosis itself is not a contraindication for return to play for athletes with otherwise normal images [44].

Traumatic Cervical Disc Herniation

Definition and Mechanism of Injury

An acute cervical disc herniation most often occurs in athletes due to excessive forced neck flexion, high-energy impact to the head, or a twisting force to the neck. It is commonly seen in many sports, such as American football, rugby, baseball, and wrestling. In a disc herniation, the nucleus pulposus protrudes through a tear in the annulus fibrosus of the intervertebral disc, possibly causing a nerve root compression, or more serious, cord compression. The nucleus pulposus contains TNF-α and other proinflammatory cytokines that can also chemically irritate surrounding tissues, causing pain. Symptoms will largely depend on the location and direction of the disc herniation.

Presentation

Typical symptoms include sudden pain, muscle spasms, limited cervical neck range of motion, radicular symptoms, paresthesias, and motor deficits. Affected athletes may prefer to hold their neck in a neutral or slightly hyperextended posture. Gentle traction may alleviate symptoms. Spurling's maneuver may reproduce the symptoms. Paracentral, or posterolateral, disc herniations will often compress or irritate nerve roots that produce clinical findings and symptoms in the neck and a single upper extremity. However, central protrusion of the nucleus pulposus into the spinal canal can lead to compression of the ventral surface of the spinal cord. This can result in a transient or even permanent spinal cord injury syndrome. A comprehensive physical examination can identify the involved level of the herniation, but an MRI will confirm the diagnosis and extent of injury.

Evaluation and Management

An MRI of the cervical spine should be obtained if an athlete experiences persistent radicular symptoms or demonstrates evidence of myelopathy. If imaging reveals cord compression with myelopathy or quadriparesis, then an emergent surgical decompression is indicated, most often through an anterior cervical discectomy and fusion. Generally, athletes without evidence of myelopathy respond well to conservative treatment. This includes relative rest, NSAIDs, oral corticosteroids, physical therapy, cervical traction, or epidural steroid injections under fluoroscopy. Physical therapy should emphasize postural retraining, McKenzie techniques, scapular retraction, and scapulothoracic stabilization [15]. If conservative measures fail or symptoms are worsening, surgical interventions can be considered, such as microforaminotomy, to widen the affected foramen and relieve pressure on the affected nerve root.

Return to Play

If no persistent neurological symptoms are present, and the athlete has full, pain-free cervical range of motion, and full strength, he or she can return to play. If an athlete requires a one-level anterior cervical discectomy and fusion (ACDF) without instrumentation or a single or multilevel posterior foraminotomies, he or she can return to contact sports participation. A relative contraindication to return to play includes athletes who have undergone a two-level subaxial cervical fusion. Absolute contraindications include a three-level cervical spine fusion or any symptomatic cervical disc herniations. However, there are varying findings with regards to the likelihood of returning to contact sports if athletes undergo surgical versus nonsurgical treatment [33].

Blunt Cerebrovascular Injuries

Definition and Mechanism of Injury

Blunt neck trauma is quite common in contact sports usually resulting in minor contusions. However, such impacts have the potential to result in serious cerebrovascular injuries. Vascular injuries have been cited in several sports, including, but not limited to, martial arts, running, tennis, and soccer [45]. The carotid and vertebral arteries are at risk for injury as a result of a traumatic fracture-subluxation or, less commonly, from direct compression. Any insult that compromises the carotid or vertebral arteries can cause a dissection, an occlusion, a thrombus, or an embolism, all of which can lead to a neurologic injury, such as a stroke. Carotid or vertebral artery dissections in sports can occur from a high-speed collision or fall that results in hyperextension and rotation of the neck, leading to tearing of the intima of the vessel [15]. Vertebral artery injury in particular may be seen with a fracture or fracture-dislocation at or above the C6 vertebra. The vertebral arteries branch off the subclavian arteries on either side of the neck, entering deep to the transverse processes at C6, and coursing superiorly in the transverse foramen of each cervical vertebra. Furthermore, excessive valsalva during weightlifting can directly injure a vessel.

Cerebrovascular injury patterns vary by sport. For example, while golfers are more likely to experience an insult to the posterior circulation, perhaps due to the rotational forces involved in their swing, weightlifters are more likely to experience an insult to the anterior circulation [45]. Although rare, it is very important that medical professionals treating athletes with neck pain consider possible involvement of the vasculature structures.

Presentation

Cerebrovascular injuries can present with various symptoms depending upon severity and location of injury. Symptoms can present immediately, or evolve over hours or days (i.e., from an occluded vessel or a thrombus that then embolized).

Injury to the carotid arteries should be suspected when symptoms such as hemiparesis, hemiplegia, hemianesthesia, dysphasia or homonymous visual field defects are present, suggesting cerebral hemispheric dysfunction.

With vertebral artery injury, symptoms may manifest as any cerebellar or brainstem syndromes. Signs such as dysarthria, emesis, vertigo, ataxia, visual field deficit, cortical blindness, and diplopia may suggest vertebrobasilar insufficiency or infarction [46].

Evaluation and Management

Prompt recognition is crucial for proper evaluation, treatment, and management. On occasion, there may be a delay in neurologic deficits after injury. An athlete with a recent history of cervical spine, head or neck injury who develops new headaches or focal neurologic deficits should undergo emergent CT or MR angiography to make the diagnosis. Treatment typically involves antiplatelet or anticoagulation medication to decrease the incidence of thrombus formation and stroke, or surgical considerations.

Return to Play

Currently, there are no published guidelines for returning to sport in an athlete with a cerebrovascular injury. Of note, relative contraindications do include athletes taking antiplatelet or anticoagulation medications.

References

1. Kucera K, Cantu R. Catastrophic sports injury research: 37th Annual Report. Published online September 27, 2020. nccsir.unc.edu.
2. 2020 Annual Report – Complete Public Version. *Spinal Cord Inj Model Syst*. 2020;NSCISC National Spinal Cord Injury Statistical Center. https://www.nscisc.uab.edu/public/2020%20Annual%20Report%20-%20Complete%20Public%20Version.pdf
3. DeVivo MJ. Causes and costs of spinal cord injury in the United States. Spinal Cord. 1997;35(12):809–13. https://doi.org/10.1038/sj.sc.3100501.
4. Chan CW, Eng JJ, Tator CH, Krassioukov A. Spinal cord injury research evidence team. Epidemiology of sport-related spinal cord injuries: a systematic review. J Spinal Cord Med. 2016;39(3):255–64. https://doi.org/10.1080/10790268.2016.1138601.
5. Cooper M, McGee K, Anderson D. Epidemiology of athletic head and neck injuries. Clin Sports Med . Published online. 2003; https://doi.org/10.1016/S0278-5919(02)00110-2.
6. Meron A, McMullen C, Laker SR, Currie D, Comstock RD. Epidemiology of cervical spine injuries in high school athletes over a ten-year period. PM R. 2018;10(4):365–72. https://doi.org/10.1016/j.pmrj.2017.09.003.
7. Deckey DG, Makovicka JL, Chung AS, et al. Neck and cervical spine injuries in National College Athletic Association Athletes: a 5-year epidemiologic study. Spine. 2020;45(1):55–64. https://doi.org/10.1097/BRS.0000000000003220.
8. Torg JS, Guille JT, Jaffe S. Injuries to the cervical spine in American football players. J Bone Joint Surg Am. 2002;84(1):112–22. https://doi.org/10.2106/00004623-200201000-00017.
9. Torg JS, Ramsey-Emrhein JA. Suggested management guidelines for participation in collision activities with congenital, developmental, or postinjury lesions involving the cervical spine. Med Sci Sports Exerc. 1997;29(7 Suppl):S256–72. https://doi.org/10.1097/00005768-199707001-00008.
10. Gianotti S, Hume PA, Hopkins WG, Harawira J, Truman R. Interim evaluation of the effect of a new scrum law on neck and back injuries in rugby union. Br J Sports Med. 2008;42(6):427–30. https://doi.org/10.1136/bjsm.2008.046987.
11. Tator CH, Carson JD, Edmonds VE. Spinal injuries in ice hockey. Clin Sports Med. 1998;17(1):183–94. https://doi.org/10.1016/s0278-5919(05)70072-7.
12. White AA, Johnson RM, Panjabi MM, Southwick WO. Biomechanical analysis of clinical stability in the cervical spine. Clin Orthop. 1975;109:85–96. https://doi.org/10.1097/00003086-197506000-00011.
13. Swartz EE, Boden BP, Courson RW, et al. National athletic trainers' association position statement: acute management of the cervical spine-

injured athlete. J Athl Train. 2009;44(3):306–31. https://doi.org/10.4085/1062-6050-44.3.306.
14. Dodwell ER, Kwon BK, Hughes B, et al. Spinal column and spinal cord injuries in mountain bikers: a 13-year review. Am J Sports Med. 2010;38(8):1647–52. https://doi.org/10.1177/0363546510365532.
15. Ramin J, Chang LG, Chang RG. Cervical Spine Injuries. In: Miranda-Comas G, Cooper G, Herrera J, Curtis S, editors. . Essential sports medicine: a clinical guide for students and residents: Springer International Publishing; 2021. p. 151–74. https://doi.org/10.1007/978-3-030-64316-4_9.
16. Aito S, D'Andrea M, Werhagen L. Spinal cord injuries due to diving accidents. Spinal Cord. 2005;43(2):109–16. https://doi.org/10.1038/sj.sc.3101695.
17. Silver JR. Spinal injuries in sports in the UK. Br J Sports Med. 1993;27(2):115–20. https://doi.org/10.1136/bjsm.27.2.115.
18. Narayana Kurup JK, Jampani R, Mohanty SP. Catastrophic cervical spinal injury in an amateur college wrestler. BMJ Case Rep. Published online July 18. 2017:bcr-2017-220260. https://doi.org/10.1136/bcr-2017-220260.
19. Kuster D, Gibson A, Abboud R, Drew T. Mechanisms of cervical spine injury in rugby union: a systematic review of the literature. Br J Sports Med. 2012;46(8):550–4. https://doi.org/10.1136/bjsports-2011-090360.
20. Nemani VM, Kim HJ. The Management of Unstable Cervical Spine Injuries. Clin Med Insights Trauma Intensive Med. 2014;5:CMTIM.S12263. https://doi.org/10.4137/CMTIM.S12263.
21. Tenny S, Varacallo M. Odontoid Fractures. In: StatPearls. StatPearls Publishing; 2021. Accessed November 11, 2021. http://www.ncbi.nlm.nih.gov/books/NBK441956/.
22. Rodts GE, Baum GR, Stewart FG, Heller JG. Motion-preserving, 2-stage transoral and posterior treatment of an unstable Jefferson fracture in a professional football player. J Neurosurg Spine. 2018;28(2):149–53. https://doi.org/10.3171/2017.6.SPINE17274.
23. Dettling SD, Morscher MA, Masin JS, Adamczyk MJ. Cranial nerve IX and X impairment after a sports-related Jefferson (C1) fracture in a 16-year-old male: a case report. J Pediatr Orthop. 2013;33(3):e23–7. https://doi.org/10.1097/BPO.0b013e3182746bc1.
24. Ferro FP, Borgo GD, Letaif OB, Cristante AF, Marcon RM, Iutaka AS. Espondilolistese traumática do áxis: epidemiologia, conduta e evolução. Acta Ortopédica Bras. 2012;20(2):84–7. https://doi.org/10.1590/S1413-78522012000200005.
25. Hsu WK, Anderson PA. Odontoid Fractures: Update on Management. Am Acad Orthop Surg. 2010;18(7):383–94. https://doi.org/10.5435/00124635-201007000-00001.

26. Bransford RJ, Alton TB, Patel AR, Bellabarba C. Upper cervical spine trauma. J Am Acad Orthop Surg. 2014;22(11):718–29. https://doi.org/10.5435/JAAOS-22-11-718.
27. Blanksby BA, Wearne FK, Elliott BC, Blitvich JD. Aetiology and occurrence of diving injuries: a review of diving safety. Sports Med. 1997;23(4):228–46. https://doi.org/10.2165/00007256-199723040-00003.
28. Langer PR, Fadale PD, Palumbo MA. Catastrophic neck injuries in the collision sport athlete. Sports Med Arthrosc Rev. 2008;16(1):7–15. https://doi.org/10.1097/JSA.0b013e318163be37.
29. Tassone JC, Duey-Holtz A. Spine concerns in the special Olympian with Down syndrome. Sports Med Arthrosc Rev. 2008;16(1):55–60. https://doi.org/10.1097/JSA.0b013e3181629ac4.
30. Concannon LG, Harrast MA, Herring SA. Radiating upper limb pain in the contact sport athlete: an update on transient quadriparesis and stingers. Curr Sports Med Rep. 2012;11(1):28–34. https://doi.org/10.1249/JSR.0b013e318240dc3f.
31. Dorshimer GW, Kelly M. Cervical pain in the athlete: common conditions and treatment. Prim Care. 2005;32(1):231–43. https://doi.org/10.1016/j.pop.2004.11.005.
32. Cantu RC. The cervical spinal stenosis controversy. Clin Sports Med. 1998;17(1):121–6. https://doi.org/10.1016/s0278-5919(05)70066-1.
33. Schroeder GD, Vaccaro AR. Cervical spine injuries in the athlete. J Am Acad Orthop Surg. 2016;24(9):e122–33. https://doi.org/10.5435/JAAOS-D-15-00716.
34. Bowles DR, Canseco JA, Alexander TD, Schroeder GD, Hecht AC, Vaccaro AR. The prevalence and Management of Stingers in college and professional collision athletes. Curr Rev Musculoskelet Med. 2020;13(6):651–62. https://doi.org/10.1007/s12178-020-09665-5.
35. Chung AS, Makovicka JL, Hassebrock JD, et al. Epidemiology of cervical injuries in NCAA football players. Spine. 2019;44(12):848–54. https://doi.org/10.1097/BRS.0000000000003008.
36. Charbonneau RME, McVeigh SA, Thompson K. Brachial neuropraxia in Canadian Atlantic university sport football players: what is the incidence of "stingers"? Clin J Sport Med. 2012;22(6):472–7. https://doi.org/10.1097/JSM.0b013e3182699ed5.
37. Kawasaki T, Ota C, Yoneda T, et al. Incidence of stingers in young Rugby players. Am J Sports Med. 2015;43(11):2809–15. https://doi.org/10.1177/0363546515597678.
38. Levitz CL, Reilly PJ, Torg JS. The pathomechanics of chronic, recurrent cervical nerve root neuropraxia. The chronic burner syndrome. Am J Sports Med. 1997;25(1):73–6. https://doi.org/10.1177/036354659702500114.

39. Meyer SA, Schulte KR, Callaghan JJ, et al. Cervical spinal stenosis and stingers in collegiate football players. Am J Sports Med. 1994;22(2):158–66. https://doi.org/10.1177/036354659402200202.
40. Kelly JD, Aliquo D, Sitler MR, Odgers C, Moyer RA. Association of burners with cervical canal and foraminal stenosis. Am J Sports Med. 2000;28(2):214–7. https://doi.org/10.1177/03635465000280021201.
41. Weinstein SM. Assessment and rehabilitation of the athlete with a "stinger". A model for the management of noncatastrophic athletic cervical spine injury. Clin Sports Med. 1998;17(1):127–35. https://doi.org/10.1016/s0278-5919(05)70067-3.
42. Ahearn BM, Starr HM, Seiler JG. Traumatic brachial plexopathy in athletes: current concepts for diagnosis and Management of Stingers. J Am Acad Orthop Surg. 2019;27(18):677–84. https://doi.org/10.5435/JAAOS-D-17-00746.
43. Weinberg J, Rokito S, Silber JS. Etiology, treatment, and prevention of athletic "stingers.". Clin Sports Med. 2003;22(3):493–500.
44. Zaremski JL, Horodyski M, Herman DC. Recurrent stingers in an adolescent American football player: dilemmas of return to play. A case report and review of the literature. Res Sports Med Print. 2017;25(3):384–90. https://doi.org/10.1080/15438627.2017.1314297.
45. Schlemm L, Nolte CH, Engelter ST, Endres M, Ebinger M. Cervical artery dissection after sports—an analytical evaluation of 190 published cases. Eur Stroke J. 2017;2(4):335–45. https://doi.org/10.1177/2396987317720544.
46. Bailes JE, Petschauer M, Guskiewicz KM, Marano G. Management of cervical spine injuries in athletes. J Athl Train. 2007;42(1):126–34.

Rheumatologic Causes of Neck Pain

German Valdez

Introduction

Rheumatic diseases are difficult to define and categorize, but generally are viewed as systemic autoimmune and inflammatory conditions which affect organs, bones, joints, and muscles. In the United States, there are approximately 11 million adults who suffer from a rheumatic disease [1] (**Rheum.org**).

In this chapter we will present various rheumatological diseases which may present with neck pain. Osteoarthritis is often categorized under rheumatic disease; for the purpose of this chapter, osteoarthritis will be excluded, and rather we will focus on autoimmune inflammatory conditions and/or diseases typically treated by rheumatologists.

Rheumatoid Arthritis

Rheumatoid arthritis (RA) is a systemic autoimmune disease characterized by chronic inflammatory synovitis. RA is the most common rheumatologic condition affecting the neck or cervical

G. Valdez (✉)
Department of Rehabilitation and Human Performance, Icahn School of Medicine at Mount Sinai, New York, NY, USA
e-mail: German.Valdez@mountsinai.org

spine [2] (**Krauss**). RA affects 1–2% of the US population and is notably three times more prevalent in women. Among all RA patients, 17–84% of patients have cervical spine disease [3] (**Kim D.H**).

Pathophysiology

Rheumatoid arthritis is believed to cause cervical spine disease when the inflammatory process extends into the neurocentral joints resulting in ligament rupture, apophyseal joint erosions, disc herniation with subsequent instability, and subluxation [4] (**Neo M**). The most commonly affected joint is the occipitoatlantoaxial junction. Atlantoaxial subluxation is a common finding, affecting nearly 90% of patients. The more common anterior subluxation is due to transverse ligament destruction, while posterior subluxations are associated with odontoid erosions and fractures.

Late in the disease process, up to 25% of patients develop subaxial subluxation due to the destruction of multiple facet joints, the interspinous ligament, and multiple disco vertebral junctions [3] (**Kim. D.H**).

A feared complication is basilar invagination, a condition in which the skull descends the cervical spine allowing an eroded odontoid to enter the foramen magnus causing compression of the brain stem or cord, or sudden death.

Presentation and Findings

Patients present with neck pain which may radiate to the occipital or temporal region. If there is neurological involvement, symptoms may include motor weakness, sensory impairments, abnormal reflexes, and spasticity.

Symptoms typically develop after 10 years of disease duration. Cervical spine disease correlates with joint erosions, active synovitis, C-reactive protein levels, rheumatoid factor positive, rheumatoid nodules, and age of onset of RA [5] (**Nguyen**).

On physical exam, there may be loss cervical spine lordosis, resistance of passive range of motion. The most common neurological findings are hyperreflexia, motor weakness, atrophy, spasticity, and gait disorders.

Management

If disease is present, imaging should be obtained every 2–3 years. Early treatment of RA is thought to slow the progression of cervical spinal disease. Prior to procedures requiring anesthesia, patients should also undergo radiographic screening. Anti-inflammatory medications, trigger point injections, and neve blocks may provide pain relief. Neck strengthening exercises are not helpful. Manipulation of the neck is contraindicated. Surgical indications include intractable pain, instability, myelopathy, or vertebral artery compromise. Most commonly a C1–C2 fusion and occipitocervical fusion is performed.

Ankylosing Spondylitis

Ankylosing spondylitis is a chronic inflammatory disease of the sacroiliac joint leading to ankylosis. Ankylosis refers to severe spinal restriction due to bony or fibrous bridging of the joints. It affects males more than females in a 2:1 ratio [6] (**Feldtkeller**).

Presentation and Findings

Ankylosing spondylitis typically presents before the age of 40 years with the most common symptom being inflammatory back pain. The pain often improves with exercise, is present at night, and improves upon arising. It often does not improve with rest. In the setting of sacroiliac involvement, there is often alternating buttock pain. In the setting of enthesitis of the supraspinatus tendon, Achilles tendon, or intercostal tendon, there may be shoulder pain, heel pain, and costochondritic chest pain, respectively. Non-musculoskeletal symptoms include symptoms from anterior uveitis, psoriasis, inflammatory bowel disease such as eye pain, visual changes, skin and nail problems, diarrhea, fever, and weight loss [7] (**Elewaut**).

In terms of the neck, similarly to rheumatoid arthritis patients may develop atlantoaxial subluxation leading to neck pain. Patients are thought to be at increased risk due to ligamentous calcification and cervical ossification. Of note, due to secondary osteopenia and osteoporosis, patients are at increased risk of spinal fractures and may develop fractures after minimal trauma.

On exam, patients will commonly have limited range of motion of the spine, SI joint tenderness, peripheral joint synovitis, enthesal tenderness. Laboratory findings include elevated CRP and is also commonly associated with HLA-B27. Imaging will reveal inflammatory sacroiliac joint inflammatory changes such as widening, erosions, sclerosis, or ankylosis [8] (**Huerta-Sil**).

Management

There is typically a long delay between 5 and 10 years between the arrival of symptoms and diagnosis. Management includes exercise, physical therapy, NSAIDS, and tumor necrosis factor (TNF) antagonists.

Diffuse Idiopathic Skeletal Hyperostosis

Diffuse idiopathic skeletal hyperostosis (DISH) is a condition characterized by calcification and ossification of spinal ligaments and entheses. The incidence of DISH increases with age and is more commonly seen in men [9] (**Belanger**). The pathogenesis of DISH is currently not well understood.

Presentation and Findings

Patients with DISH most commonly present with thoracic back pain, but may also present with neck pain, low back pain, or extremity pain. Roughly 80% of patients will present with morning back stiffness. Involvement of the cervical spine often presents with dysphagia, but may also present with hoarseness, stridor, aspiration pneumonia, sleep apnea, atlantoaxial subluxation, or thoracic outlet syndrome [10] (**Mader**). More serious complications such as spinal cord compression may arise when there is involvement of the posterior longitudinal ligament.

On physical exam, patients commonly have decreased range of motion of thoracic lateral flexion, along with tenderness and/or palpable nodules over entheses. The palpable nodules are typically found over the calcaneus, olecranon, and patella.

Diagnosis of DISH is made via radiographic imaging. Hallmark findings include ossification of the paravertebral ligament and peripheral entheses. In addition, imaging will often reveal linear calcification and ossification along the anterolateral aspect of vertebral bodies [11] (**Forestier**).

Management

Treatment is aimed at symptomatic relief and maintaining function. Pain is often addressed with Acetaminophen or NSAIDs while function is addressed with range of motion and stretching exercises [12] (**Al-Herz**). Surgery may be warranted to remove bony spurs leading to the more severe complications such as dysphagia and myelopathy.

Myositis

Dermatomyositis and polymyositis are both inflammatory myopathies with a prevalence of 1 per 100,000 and is more commonly seen in woman in a 2:1 ratio.

Presentation and Findings

Patients typically present with gradually worsening proximal muscle weakness. Commonly including muscles of the trunk, shoulders and upper arms, thighs, and neck extensors. Due to the weakness patients will often report difficulty brushing their hair, rising from chair, and walking uphill [13] (**Harris Love**). Patients may also present with myalgias, which may include the neck. In dermatomyositis patients also present with distinct skin rashes. Laboratory findings include an elevated creatine kinase.

In both the conditions, physical exam may reveal mechanic's hand; i.e., thickened cracked skin at the tips and lateral aspect of the fingers and palm [14] (**Sunkureddi**).

In dermatomyositis, physical exam may reveal as a violaceous or erythematous scaly rash over extensor surfaces of the elbows, knees, and the MCP and IP joints, also known as Gottron papules. Skin findings also include a heliotrope rash with periorbital edema, and the shawl sign, a diffuse erythematous rash over the chest and shoulder in a shawl-like distribution.

Laboratory findings include elevated muscle enzymes such as creatine kinase, lactate dehydrogenase, aldolase, aspartate aminotransferase, alanine aminotransferase. Other abnormal labs which may be found are anti-Sm, SS-A, SS-B, antiribonucleoprotein, and anti-Jo-1.

Management

Treatment includes corticosteroids and other immunosuppressive agents such as methotrexate, azathioprine, cyclosporine, cyclophosphamide, rituximab, mycophenolate mofetil, rituximab, TNF antagonist, and high-dose IVIG.

Fibromyalgia

Fibromyalgia is described as a nonprogressive diffuse pain syndrome of unknown cause associated with multiple tender points. Fibromyalgia affects 1–4% of the population, with roughly 75% of patients being female [15] (**Weir**).

Presentation and Findings

Patients often present with diffuse body pain including the neck and the bilateral upper and lower extremities. Pain is often migratory and waxes and wanes in intensity. Along with pain, patients commonly present with fatigue and sleep disturbances [16] (**Bellato**).

On physical exam, patients will have 11 of 18 tender points as described by the American College of Rheumatology, otherwise the musculoskeletal and neurological physical exams are unremarkable.

Management

Treatment of fibromyalgia includes education of the condition, aerobic exercise, cognitive behavioral therapy, stress management, optimizing sleep hygiene, and pharmacologic therapy. Psychotropic agents such as tricyclic antidepressants, serotonin reuptake inhibitors, and norepinephrine serotonin reuptake inhibitors have all shown to be efficacious. Other efficacious agents include anticonvulsants, gabapentin, and pre-gabalin.

Conclusion

Although not as common as conditions previously discussed in this book, systemic rheumatological conditions may also be responsible for neck pain. Clinical suspicion for these illnesses is critical as the correct diagnosis will dictate proper management.

References

1. American College of Rheumatology. https://www.rheumatology.org/Portals/0/Files/ACR-COVID-19-Clinical-Guidance-Summary-Patients-with-Rheumatic-Diseases.pdf.

2. Krauss WE, Bledsoe JM, Clarke MJ, et al. Rheumatoid arthritis of the cranio-vertebral junction. Neurosurgery. 2010;66:83–95.
3. Kim DH, Hilibrand AS. Rheumatoid arthritis in the cervical spine. J Am Acad Orthop Surg. 2005;13:463–74.
4. Neo M. Treatment of upper cervical spine involvement in rheumatoid arthritis patients. Mod Rheumatol. 2008;18:327–35.
5. Nguyen HV, Ludwing SC, Solber JK, et al. Rheumatoid arthritis of the cervical spine. Spine J. 2004;4:329–34.
6. Feldtkeller E, Khan MA, van der Heijde D, et al. Age at disease onset and diagnosis delay in HLAB27 negative vs. positive patients with ankylosing spondylitis. Rheumatol Int. 2003;23:61–6.
7. Elewaut D, Matucci-Cerinic M. Treatment of ankylosing spondylitis and extra-articular manifestations in everyday rheumatology practice. Rheumatology (Oxford). 2009;48:1029–35.
8. Huerta-Sil G, Casasola-Vargas JC, Londona JD, et al. Low grade radiographic sacroiliitis as prognostic factor in patients with undifferentiated spondyloarthritis fulfilling diagnostic criteria for ankylosing spondylitis throughout follow up. Ann Rheum Dis. 2006;65:642–6.
9. Belanger TA, Rowe DE. Diffuse idiopathic skeletal hyperostosis: musculoskeletal manifestations. J Am Acad Orthop Surg. 2001;9:258–67.
10. Mader R. Clinical manifestations of diffuse idiopathic skeletal hyperostosis of the cervical spine. Semin Arthritis Rheum. 2002;32:130–2.
11. Forestier J, Lagier R. Ankylosing hyperostosis of the spine. Clin Orthop Relat Res. 1971;74:65–83.
12. Al-Herz A, Snip JP, Clark B, et al. Exercise therapy for patients with diffuse idiopathic skeletal hyperostosis. Clin Rheumatol. 2008;27:207–10.
13. Harris-Love MO, Shrader JA, Koziol D, et al. Distribution and severity of weakness among patients with polymyositis, dermatomyositis and juvenile dermatomyositis. Rheumatology (Oxford). 2009;48:134–9.
14. Sunkureddi P, Nguyen-Oghalai T, Jarvis J, et al. Clinical signs of dermatomyositis. Hosp Physician. 2005;41:41–4.
15. Weir PT, Harlan GA, Nkoy FL, et. al. The incidence of fibromyalgia and its associated comorbidities: a population-based retrospective cohort study based on International Classification of Diseases, 9th Revision codes. J Clin Rheumatol. 2006;12:124–8.
16. Bellato E, Marini E, Castoldi F, et al. Fibromyalgia syndrome: etiology, pathogenesis, diagnosis, and treatment [published correction appears in Pain Res Treat. 2013;2013:960270]. Pain Res Treat. 2012;2012:426130. https://doi.org/10.1155/2012/426130.

Case Studies

Caroline Varlotta

Case 1: Cervical Spondylosis

A 72-year-old male presents to the office with a chief complaint of neck pain for 30 years. He denies numbness or tingling in his upper extremities. He reports restricted range of motion and increased pain with physical exercise and sitting at a computer. He has experienced progressive difficulty turning his head left and right while driving. He has history of lumbar laminectomy, psoriasis, hypertension, diabetes, hyperlipidemia, cholecystectomy, and prostatectomy. He also reports multiple sports injuries when playing football in high school with "stingers and burners" and two motor vehicle accidents. His occupation is a lawyer. His BMI is 35 kg/m^2.

On exam, the patient has forward head position, with his external auditory meatus 3 inches anterior to the acromioclavicular joint, and a thoracic kyphosis. He has psoriasis plaques on elbows. He has bilateral restricted range of motion in the cervical spine with extension, side bending, and rotation. He has pain with joint/plane motions at C4/5, C5/6, and C6/7. He has full strength in his

---

C. Varlotta (✉)
Department of Rehabilitation and Human Performance, Icahn School of Medicine at Mount Sinai, New York, NY, USA

bilateral upper extremities. Deep tendon reflexes are 2+. His sensation is intact. Spurling, Lhermitte, Tinel at elbow and wrist, and Adson's are negative. On functional evaluation, he has normal toe and heel walking, normal balance, and normal tandem.

X-ray demonstrated C4/C5 and C5/C6 spondylosis, loss of intervertebral disc height, and osteophyte formation in the uncovertebral joints. In the thoracic spine, there is evidence of disc degeneration with Scheuermann's kyphosis. There were no arthritic changes noted in the SI joint on lumbar X-ray. MRI findings were consistent with degenerative disc disease, no evidence of central stenosis, and mild to moderate foraminal stenosis at multiple levels (Figs. 9.1 and 9.2).

The patient was diagnosed with multilevel cervical spondylosis with hyper-lordosis, cervical facet arthropathy, thoracic disc degeneration with Scheuermann's kyphosis, and possible psoriatic arthritis.

Medications prescribed include NSAIDs and Flexeril 10 mg at night. He was referred to physical therapy and for weight loss management. He was advised on ergonomic activity modification. He underwent cervical intraarticular facet joint injection with relief.

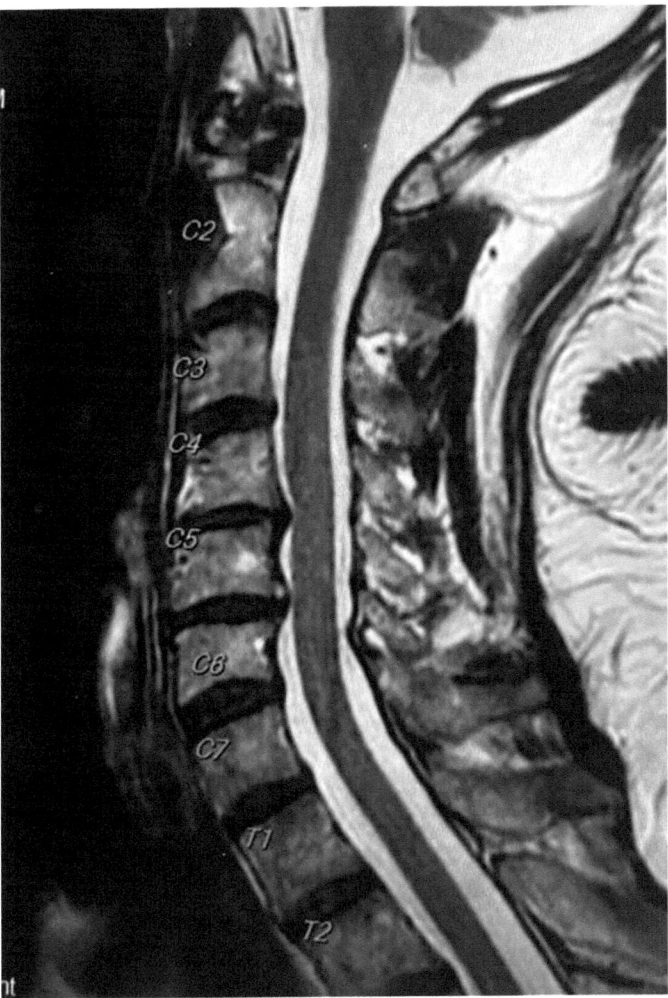

Fig. 9.1 MRI in sagittal view of cervical spondylosis with right greater than left foraminal stenosis at C4/C5 and C5/C6, central spinal stenosis, decreased intervertebral disc height

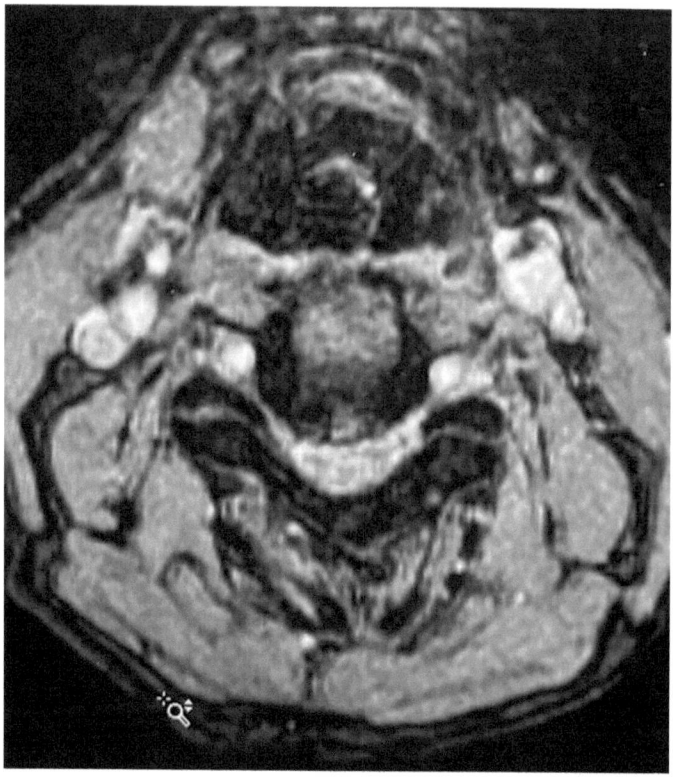

Fig. 9.2 MRI axial view of cervical spondylosis

Case 2: Cervical Myelopathy

A 65-year-old woman presents with one and a half years of neck discomfort associated with restricted range of motion. One year ago, she had onset of numbness and tingling in the bilateral fourth and fifth fingers and the bottoms of her feet. This sensation does not affect her sleep and are not exacerbated with physical activities. She denies weakness, history of trauma, or prior neck surgery. However, the patient reports loss of balance on occasion, which has worsened over the past year. She reports no falls and no difficulty swallowing. Medical history includes unilateral laryngeal atrophy with vocal cord dysfunction and mild hyperlipidemia.

On exam, she has bilateral restricted range of motion in the cervical spine with side bending and rotation. Sensation and motor are intact throughout. Deep tendon reflexes are brisk (3+) throughout. Spurling and Hoffman are mildly positive, and Babinski, Tinel at the elbow and wrist, Allen, Adson, and Phalen's tests are all negative. Lhermitte's test is positive. She has no clonus. Toe walking, heel walking, one legged stance, and tandem are consistent with mild vestibular dysfunction.

X-ray of the cervical spine demonstrates straightening of the cervical lordosis with C5/C6 and C6/C7 spondylosis associated with loss of intravertebral disc height. There is no evidence of pannus formation or C1/C2 instability. Flexion and extension views demonstrate no evidence of transitory motion. Oblique views have evidence of mild foraminal stenosis.

MRI of the cervical spine demonstrates moderate to severe cervical stenosis from C5 to C7 associated with loss of intervertebral disc height. There is moderate foraminal stenosis at C5/C6 and C6/C7 bilaterally. Additionally, there is anterior and posterior compression of the spinal cord with gliosis (Fig. 9.3). Electromyography (EMG) has no evidence of cervical radiculopathy or compressive neuropathy.

The patient was diagnosed with cervical spondylosis from C5 to C7 with moderate to severe stenosis and myeloradiculopathy. She is advised to follow neurological precautions with activities. Pharmacologic treatment includes Medrol dose pack, gabapentin 300 mg TID, and meloxicam. Physical therapy is focused on strengthening and balance, with cervical spine and neurologic precautions, which includes no cervical traction or manipulation. Injections are not initially indicated in this patient due to the spinal cord compression. Surgical consultations include orthopedic spine and neurosurgery. Her options regarding surgery include observation, posterior laminectomy or laminoplasty, and anterior cervical decompression and fusion from C5 to C7, likely accessing on the side of the laryngeal atrophy.

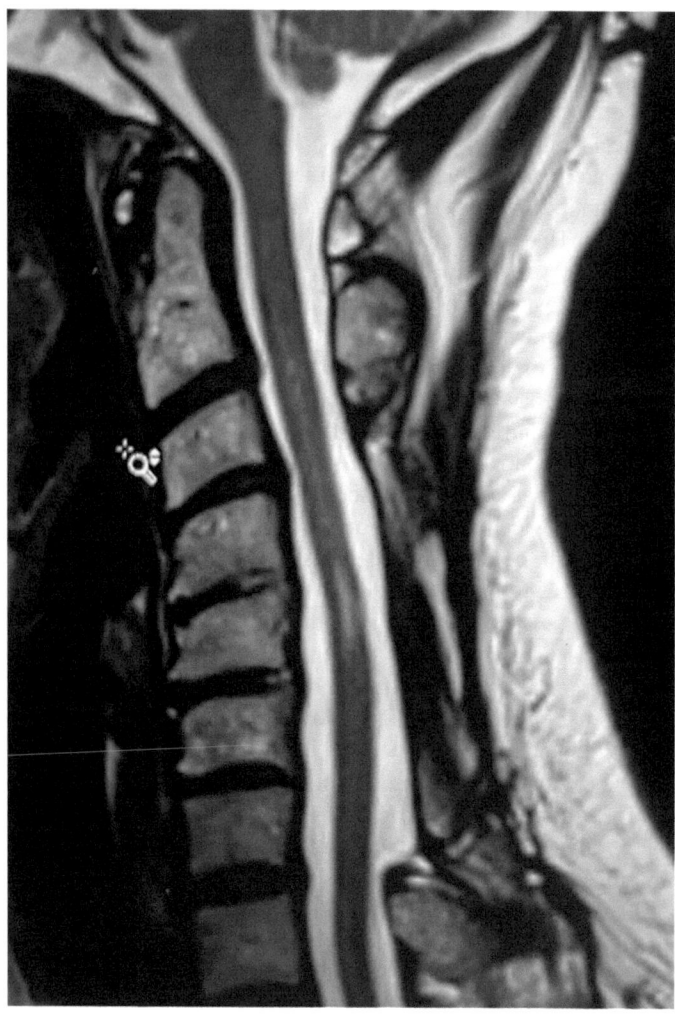

Fig. 9.3 MRI sagittal view of cervical spondylosis C4–C7 with myelomalacia at C5–C6

Case 3: Cervical Dystonia

A 33-year-old female graphic designer presents with 10-year history of neck discomfort associated with headache. She reports failing multiple treatments with a previous physician, including medications, physical therapy, chiropractor, acupuncture, and massage. Trigger point injections provided temporary pain relief. Her pain is interfering with work, as she cannot sit at a computer for prolonged periods of time due to increased neck spasms. It is also interfering with sleep. She has history of ADHD, is on Adderall, and history of anxiety and depression, on Wellbutrin and Lexapro. There are no changes in the pain with menstruation or physical activity. Imaging 5 years ago revealed no evidence of degenerative changes in the cervical spine.

On exam, the patient has postural kyphosis. She has full range of motion of her neck and upper extremities but has evidence of hypermobility and multidirectional instability of bilateral shoulders. Her distal strength is intact. However, she has 4/5 weakness in her periscapular muscles and rotator cuff and shoulder subluxation without labral click. Sensation, reflexes, and functional evaluation are normal. She has trigger points in her cervical paraspinal muscles, trapezius, and sternocleidomastoid bilaterally, with evidence of TMJ. Adson's, Tinel's, and Roos tests are negative.

Cervical and thoracic radiographs are ordered to assess for interval changes since prior imaging. Cervical spine X-ray demonstrated no degenerative changes but straightening of cervical lordosis. Thoracic X-ray demonstrated mild postural kyphoscoliosis. MRI of the cervical spine has no evidence of disc degeneration nor neural compression.

The patient was diagnosed with cervical dystonia, hypermobility syndrome, postural kyphoscoliosis, and bilateral shoulder subluxation.

Her treatment plan included pharmacologic management with NSAIDs, topical Lidoderm patch, diclofenac topical gel, Lyrica 50 mg, titrated to 300 mg daily, and continuation of current antidepressant mediations, with consideration to change to Cymbalta or duloxetine. She was referred to physical therapy for stretching, strengthening, and postural control, and she was prescribed a postural control brace and home neuromuscular electrical stimulation unit (Fig. 9.4, from Google Images). Consult was placed for a dentist for treatment of TMJ with oral orthotic. No surgical referrals were placed. If her symptoms do not resolve, she may be a candidate for Botox injections for cervical dystonia.

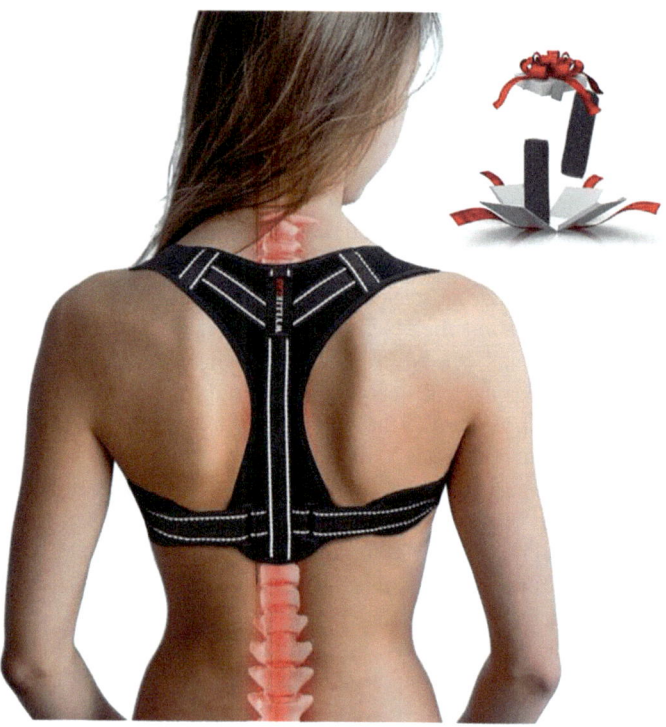

Fig. 9.4 Postural control brace

Case 4: Cervical Herniation with Radiculopathy

A 52-year-old engineer presents with 2 weeks of severe neck and right arm pain, associated with difficulty extending his head, weakness in right upper extremity, and impaired sleep. The pain initially started 2 months prior in Texas when the patient was working on a project erecting tents for undocumented migrants. At that time, the pain manifested as mild discomfort in the cervical spine with radiation into right interscapular region. He was evaluated in urgent care 2 weeks ago when his symptoms became so severe and he was unable to work. At urgent care, he was prescribed ibuprofen 800 mg, dosed, Toradol 30 mg injection, and given a cervical spine soft collar. He reports no history of trauma.

He presents on exam with forward flexed posture and torticollis. Pain is exacerbated with sidebending right, rotating right, and with extension. Deep tendon reflexes and sensation are normal. Muscle strength is diminished in the right upper extremity, specifically the deltoid, biceps, and rhomboids are only anti-gravity. Apley's compression test and Spurling's test are positive on the right.

The patient brought his X-ray from urgent care, which revealed C5/6 degeneration with loss of intervertebral disc height, and focal kyphosis at C4/5. An MRI of the cervical spine was ordered, which revealed a right-sided far lateral and foraminal herniated disc at C5/6 with compression of the C6 nerve root (Figs. 9.5 and 9.6).

The diagnosis was right C5/C6 foraminal herniated disc with right C6 radiculopathy. Pharmacologic treatment included Medrol dose pack, and gabapentin 300 mg TID, which was titrated up to 600 mg TID. Analgesics were ordered for as needed. He was referred to orthopedic spine surgery for microscopic discectomy and nerve decompression without fusion, and for a postoperative rehabilitation program.

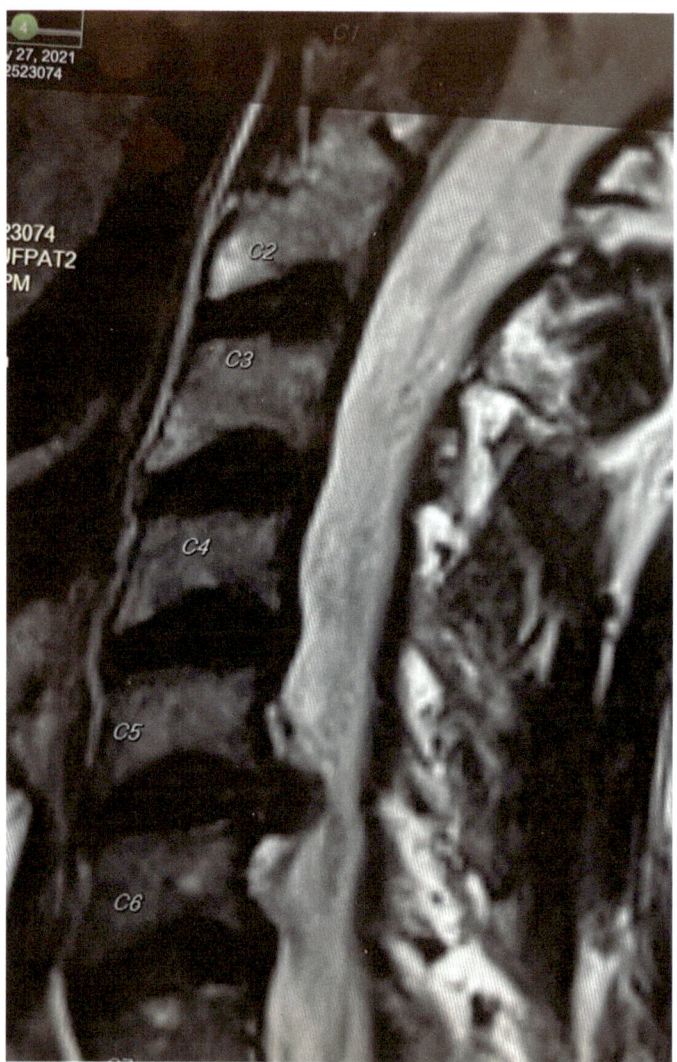

Fig. 9.5 MRI parasagittal view of herniated disc C5/C6

9 Case Studies

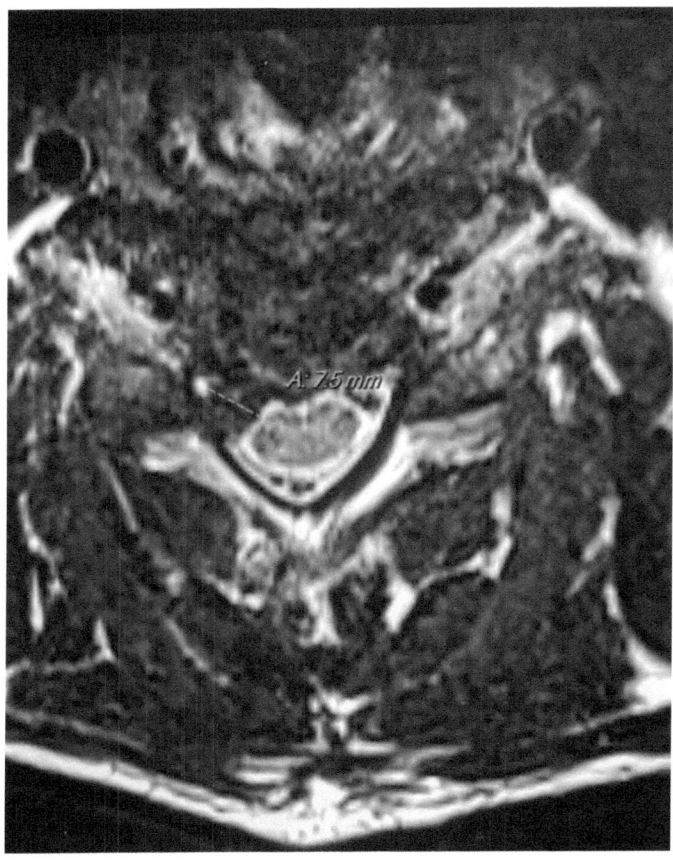

Fig. 9.6 MRI axial view of herniated disc C5/C6

Index

A
Acceleration-deceleration injury, 18, 19
Acetaminophen, 43
Achondroplasia, 69
Aditya, R., 65
Afifi, T., 65
Aito, S., 99
Anesthesia, 82
Ankylosing spondylitis, 121, 122
Annulus fibrosis (AF), 38
Anterior atlantoaxial subluxation (AAS), 75
Anterior cervical discectomy and fusion (ACDF), 112
Anticonvulsants, 44
Apley's compression test, 135
Atlantoaxial instability, 75
Atypical cervical vertebrae, 3

B
Blunt cerebrovascular injuries, 112–113
Blunt neck trauma, 112
Brachial plexus, 10
Burst fracture, 98

C
Calcification of the ligamentum flavum (CLF), 74
Cartilaginous endplate (EP), 38
Catastrophic spinal injuries, 95

Cell therapy, 45
Central cord syndrome, 99
Cerebrovascular injury, 113
Cervical axial pain, 17
Cervical cord neurapraxia (CCN), 105–107
Cervical dermatomes, 29
Cervical disc herniation (CDH), 45, 72
Cervical dystonia, 133–135
Cervical facet joint syndrome, *see* Facet joint syndrome
Cervical herniation with radiculopathy, 135–137
Cervical lymphatic system, 14
Cervical muscles, 5, 7
Cervical myelopathy, 42, 130–131
    CDH, 72
    cervical spinal stenosis, 66
    cervical spine anomalies, 76, 77
    CLF, 74
    CSM, 71
    DCM, 70
    definition, 65
    demographic of patients, 69, 70
    diagnostic approach, 82–84
    differential diagnosis, 84, 85
    DSA, 76
    etiologies, 67, 68
    myelomalacia, 66
    OLF, 74
    OPLL, 73
    pathophysiology, 77–78
    patient's history, 79
    physical exam, 79–82
    prognosis, 87–88
    rheumatoid arthritis, 74
    risk factors, 67–69
    signs and symptoms, 78–79
    spinal tumors, 75–76
    treatment, 86–87
    treatment and management, 84–87
Cervical neurologic injury, 107
Cervical OPLL, 73
Cervical plexus, 10
Cervical radiculopathy
    anatomy, 56
    clinical presentation, 57, 58
    diagnosis, 58, 59
    epidemiology, 56
    management, 60
    mechanism of injury, 57
    outcomes, 61

Cervical spinal stenosis, 66
Cervical spine, 2
Cervical spine anomalies, 76, 77
Cervical spine radiographs (X-Rays), 83
Cervical spondylosis, 71, 127–129
Cervical spondylotic myelopathy (CSM), 66, 71, 88
Cervical strains and sprains
  epidemiology, 17, 18
  history, 19
  imaging, 20
  pathophysiology, 18, 19
  pharmacotherapy, 20, 21
  physical examination, 20
  physical modalities, 21, 22
Cervical subcutaneous tissue, 4
Cervical sympathetic ganglia, 11
Cervical transverse processes, 3
Cervical vertebrae, 2–4
Cervicothoracic stabilization exercises, 21, 22
Collagen type I alpha1 gene (COLIA1), 40
Collagen type II alpha2 gene (COL11A2), 40
Congenital spinal anomalies, 104
Congenital stenosis, 69
Costocervical trunk, 13
Craniocervical junction (CCJ), 2
Cyclobenzaprine, 44
Cymbalta, 134

D

Deep cervical fascia, 4
Deep cervical flexor muscles, 6
Degenerative cervical myelopathy (DCM), 66, 70
Degenerative disc disease (DDD), 47, 72
Demyelination, 67
Dermatomyositis, 123, 124
Destructive spondyloarthropathy (DSA), 76
Dialysis-related spondyloarthropathy (DRSA), 76
Diffuse idiopathic skeletal hyperostosis (DISH), 73, 122, 123
Diffusion tensor imaging, 83
Disc degeneration, 39, 40
Discectomy, 87
Discogenic pain
  biomechanics/pathophysiology, 38, 40, 41
  clinical presentation, 41, 42
  imaging, 42, 43
  non-operative treatment, 43, 44
  operative treatment, 45–47

Discography, 43
Dodwell, E.R., 101
Dorsal root ganglion (DRG), 9
Down syndrome (DS), 76, 104
Duloxetine, 134
Dynamic stabilization, 47

E
Edema, 67
Ehlers-Danlos syndrome, 104
Electrodiagnostic testing (EDX), 109
Electromyography (EMG), 131
Epidural injections, 44
Erector spinae muscles, 6

F
Facet joint degeneration, 27
Facet joint dislocations, 99, 100
Facet joint syndrome
   anatomy, 26, 27
   clinical presentation, 28
   diagnosis, 31, 32
   differential diagnosis, 32
   epidemiology, 25, 26
   pathophysiology, 27
   physical examination, 28
      cervical Kemp's test, 31
      inspection, 28
      motor testing, 30
      palpation, 29
      range of motion, 29
      reflexes, 30
      sensory testing, 30
      spring test, 31
   treatment, 33
Farfan, H.F., 38
Fibrodysplasia ossificans, 76
Fibromyalgia, 124, 125
Flexion teardrop fracture, 98
Foraminotomy, 87
Freedman, R., 95

G

Gene polymorphisms, 40
Gene therapy, 44
Ghazzi, M., 2, 4, 5, 8, 9, 12–14
Goldenhar syndrome, 76, 77
Gottron papules, 124

H

Ha, K.-Y., 26
Harbus, M., 2, 4, 5, 8, 9, 12–14, 17–19, 21, 22, 55, 56, 58, 59, 61, 62
Hyperextension injury, 18
Hypesthesia, 82

I

Inferior articular process, 26
Inferior cervical ganglion, 11
Inflammatory cascade, 40
Inflammatory chemical process, 57
Interspinous distraction, 46
Intervertebral disc (IVD), 37
Intradural extramedullary (IDEM) tumors, 75

J

Japanese Orthopaedic Association (JOA) classification system, 86, 87
Jefferson fracture, 101
Juvenile rheumatoid arthritis, 104

K

Kalbian, I., 95
Kirkaldy-Willis, W.H., 38
Klippel-Feil syndrome (KFS), 69, 76, 77, 104
Kniest syndrome, 76

L

Laminectomy, 87
Laminoplasty, 87
Larsen syndrome, 77
Lee, J., 55, 56, 58, 59, 61, 62

Levator scapulae muscle, 5
Loebel, 101
Lymphatics, 14

M
Marfan syndrome, 104
Matrix degrading enzymes, 40
Meninges, 8, 9
Middle cervical ganglion, 11
Morquio disease, 77
Morquio syndrome, 76
Muscle relaxants, 20, 21, 44
Myelomalacia, 66
Myofascial pain syndrome (MPS), 18, 19

N
Neck Disability Index questionnaire, 42
Neck pain, 75
Nerve roots, 9
NSAIDs, 43
Nucleus pulposus (NP), 38
Nucleus pulposus replacement, 46
Nurick grading system, 87
Nurick scale, 81

O
Obesity, 26
Odontoid fractures, 101
Odontoid process, 2
Opioids, 44
Os odontoideum, 104
Ossification of the ligamentum flavum (OLF), 74
Ossification of the posterior longitudinal ligament (OPLL), 72–73
Osteoarthritis, 27, 119

P
Paresthesia, 82
Patel, C., 25, 27–33
Phrenic nerves, 11
Polymyositis, 123
Posterior longitudinal ligament (PLL), 72
Prominens, 3

R
Ranawat Classification, 75
Rheumatic diseases
    ankylosing spondylitis, 121, 122
    dermatomyositis, 123, 124
    DISH, 122, 123
    fibromyalgia, 124, 125
    rheumatoid arthritis, 119–121
Rheumatoid arthritis (RA), 69, 74, 119–121
Roos tests, 133

S
Scalene muscles, 5, 6
Shahgholi, L., 17–19, 21, 22
Silverberg, C., 2, 4, 5, 8, 9, 12–14
Simons, D.G., 19
Soft disc herniation, 72
Soft tissue, 4
Soft tissue pain disorders, 18
Spinal cord, 7, 8
Spinal cord injuries (SCI), 96
Spinal tumors, 75–76
Spine biomechanics, 37
Spine degeneration, 38
Spondylosis, 41, 42
Sports trauma and fractures
    blunt cerebrovascular injuries, 112–113
    burst fracture, 98
    CCN, 105–107
    cervical spinous process fractures, 103
    congenital spinal anomalies, 104
    epidemiology, 96–97
    facet joint dislocations, 99, 100
    flexion teardrop fracture, 98
    hangman's fracture, 101–103
    Jefferson fracture, 101
    odontoid fractures, 101
    stinger/burners, 107–110
    traumatic cervical disc herniation, 110–112
    unstable fractures and dislocation, 97–103
    wedge fractures, 103, 104
Spurling's test, 135
Stellate ganglion, 11
Sternocleidomastoid muscle (SCM), 5

Steroids, 44
Stingers, 107
Subacromial peripheral impingement syndrome (SIAS), 56
Subaxial spine, 2
Subclavian arteries, 12
Suboccipital muscles, 7
Superior articular process, 26
Superior cervical ganglion, 11
Sympathetic trunks, 11

T
Tetreault, L.A., 67
Three joint complex, 27
Thyrocervical trunk, 13
Tizanidine, 44
Torg, J.S., 100, 103, 106
Torg-Pavlov ratio, 106
Total disc replacement (TDR), 46
Trapezius muscle, 5
Traumatic cervical disc herniation, 110–112
Travell, J.G., 18
Trentman, C., 55, 56, 58, 59, 61, 62
Tricyclic antidepressants, 44
Trisomy 21, 69
Tumor necrosis factor (TNF) antagonists, 122
Tylenol, 43

V
Vagus nerve, 10
Valdez, G., 119
Varlotta, C., 38–42, 44, 45, 47, 127
Vascular injuries, 112
Vasculature
   costocervical trunk, 13
   lymphatics, 14
   subclavian arteries, 12
   thyrocervical trunk, 13
   veins, 13
   vertebral arteries, 12
Veins, 13
Vertebral arteries, 12
Vertebral artery injury, 113
Viral infections, 85
Vitamin-D receptor (VDR), 40

W

Wallerian degeneration, 67
Wedge fractures, 103, 104
Whiplash injuries, 18, 19
Work-related cervical pain, 18

Z

Zekster, K., 65
Zygapophyseal/apophyseal joints, *see* Facet joint syndrome

GPSR Compliance

The European Union's (EU) General Product Safety Regulation (GPSR) is a set of rules that requires consumer products to be safe and our obligations to ensure this.

If you have any concerns about our products, you can contact us on ProductSafety@springernature.com

In case Publisher is established outside the EU, the EU authorized representative is:

Springer Nature Customer Service Center GmbH
Europaplatz 3
69115 Heidelberg, Germany

Batch number: 08823212

Printed by Printforce, the Netherlands